THE GODDESS PATH

13 Steps to Becoming
Your Most Intuitive,
Authentic and Powerful Self

KIRSTY GALLAGHER

Rider/Happy Place Books, an imprint of Ebury Publishing
20 Vauxhall Bridge Road
London SW1V 2SA

Rider is part of the Penguin Random House group of companies
whose addresses can be found at global.penguinrandomhouse.com

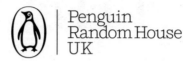

Author photo on page 257 © Alexandra Cameron

First published by Rider/Happy Place Books in 2024

www.penguin.co.uk

A CIP catalogue record for this book is available from the British Library

ISBN 9781846047763

Typeset in 11/16 pt Baskerville MT Pro by Jouve (UK), Milton Keynes
Printed and bound in Great Britain by Clays Ltd, Elcograf S.p.A.

The authorised representative in the EEA is Penguin Random House Ireland,
Morrison Chambers, 32 Nassau Street, Dublin D02 YH68

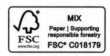

Penguin Random House is committed to a sustainable future
for our business, our readers and our planet. This book is made from
Forest Stewardship Council® certified paper.

THE GODDESS PATH

To the Goddess.

CONTENTS

'It's time to become your most powerful, magical, intuitive, liberated and wise Goddess self.'

INTRODUCTION
THE GODDESS PATH

Welcome to the Goddess Path.

This book will take you on a journey of inner exploration and self-discovery. It will help you to reawaken the Goddess within you and, in doing so, reclaim all of who you came here to be.

I started my journey with the Goddess almost 20 years ago when I went on a course to learn how to read Goddess oracle cards. I had been on a journey of spiritual discovery and exploration for a few years and was already working with Angels and subsequently angel cards. As soon as I was sent the details of this course, it felt like something I was meant to do – the natural next step. I can't explain the feeling I had – it was like a deep inner calling. The course was in London and I was living up north at the time with no idea how I'd get myself to London to do it, but I just knew that I had to go. Looking back now, I know the Goddess called me.

The course opened up a whole world of feminine wisdom and guidance that I could call on for support anytime I needed it. The comfort I found in the Goddesses was so incredible that I started incorporating the practice into my daily rituals and began to pick a card a day, leading me to work with the energies of that Goddess, exploring more of her energy, story and how she showed up in my life. It suddenly felt like I was no longer alone, and I found myself not only calling on the Goddesses for support when I needed it, but also starting to embody her qualities and feeling her energy awakening something within me.

My relationship with the Goddess and the feminine deepened in 2009 when I lived in India for a year studying yoga. Here I began to delve into daily rituals with the Goddess and learn about how we can invite her into our daily lives and, in doing so, awaken the Goddess within. I learned mantras and prayers, visited temples and devoted my life to her, the Goddess, the divine feminine. It was also during this time when I started to live alongside the moon (which is the feminine energy of the universe) and this invited me to tap much more into my own feminine flow, emotions, intuition and inner knowing, enabling me to fully connect to, awaken and embrace my own seasons, cycles, rhythms and inner Goddess.

Over the decades, I have studied many different modalities with many different teachers, but my biggest teacher has been the Goddess herself. Walking alongside her, embodying her, devoting to her has changed me and my life in ways that I can't even explain. She has helped me to know who I am, what I want and to trust myself and my emotions, intuition and innate wisdom. She has helped me to find my self-worth, claim my boundaries and discover more of my purpose. She has taught me how to awaken my sacred self and tap into the creative life force energy of the universe to create and weave and flow with life. She has freed me to become all of who I came here to be and be able to truly hear the whispers of my heart and soul.

Since I invited the Goddess into my life 20 years ago, my life has never been the same, and now I want to share with you the journey that I've been on and all that I have learned so that you too can invite the Goddess into your life and reap the endless benefits.

You are reading this book because you heard the call – the nudge that urged you to pick this book off the shelf or order it online. Or perhaps it was the little something that stirred within when you saw the beautiful front cover and you felt like the Goddess was speaking to you. This was her wanting to make herself known to you and take you on this journey of self-discovery and becoming your most powerful, magical, intuitive, liberated and wise Goddess self.

We are at a time in history right now where Goddess energy is needed more than ever. In a world gripped by the shadow masculine energies of greed, corruption, capitalism, power and control, we need to allow the feminine to rise to bring back balance.

As each one of us remembers and reclaims the Goddess within, we become part of this revolution and awakening that is so needed in the world today.

The words you read here are not mine; they are hers, yours, ours. They are the words of every woman who has gone before us and every woman yet to come who needs to hear these words and reclaim the Goddess within.

This book is a call home, to yourself and all of who you came here to be. This book is a remembering. A reclamation.

Why 13 Chapters?

This book is written as a 13-step journey; 13 chapters for you to reclaim yourself.

Firstly, I'd love to talk about why I've structured my book in 13 chapters. We all know the superstitions about the number 13, but it is an important part of our reclamation. Thirteen is the number long associated with the divine feminine, as it corresponds to the number of lunar and menstrual cycles in a year.

You may not know this, but Friday is also connected to the feminine as it was named after the Nordic Goddess Freya, or Frigg, who was the wife of Odin and the Goddess of love, marriage, fertility, sex, magic and predicting the future. In astrology, Friday is the day of the planet Venus, a day to celebrate romance, beauty and love.

At one point in time, both the number 13 and Friday were celebrated and considered to bring good fortune, and the Goddesses were even worshipped. But as the Christian church gained momentum in the Middle Ages, paganism didn't fit the agenda, particularly the worship of the menstrual cycle, fertility or Goddesses promoting unholy things such as sex, pleasure and magic. The Church went to great lengths to distance itself from these things, branding anyone who worshipped any of these things 'witches', and so began the superstition around the number 13 and Friday the 13th.

As part of walking the Goddess Path, we need to reclaim these ancient rituals, rites and Goddesses, and so we walk the path of the 13 steps to reclaim the Goddess.

The Journey You're About to Embark On

The journey through the first six chapters begins with the descent, into your depths, into the underworld, beneath the surface into all your doubts and fears, and everything that's kept you hidden, scared and small.

We then spend some time in the underworld and meet the Dark Goddess who will help you to face and embrace your shadows, search your soul and transform your life, breaking free and liberating all of you.

Taking all that you've learned and reclaimed, you then begin to ascend, through the final six chapters, remembering and reclaiming more and more of you and allowing the Goddess within to rise.

Although we call this the 'Goddess Path', I want you to remember that the feminine, the Goddess, is not linear – in the same way that the spiritual journey and the journey of life is not linear. Just like nature, the Goddess weaves, flows and spirals, and I'd love you to see this journey, and your life, as cyclical.

We don't go from A to B and everything is fixed and healed. Very often on a self-discovery or spiritual journey, there can be upset and confusion when the same things keep coming back around again. But in truth this is how we learn and grow.

On this journey you will go through seasons and cycles. You will come to realise that life will keep giving us the same lessons over and over again until we fully learn them. But as we grow and evolve on our journey, and we spiral through the same lessons and begin to deal with them differently, we don't touch quite the same depth of emotion, pain and angst each time. It's a wonderful moment along your path when you realise that had that same thing happened six months ago, you'd have dealt with it differently – this is when you know that you are growing.

See this path as a journey, a spiral. Each time you go through a lesson, a challenge and a period of growth, it's bringing you back into your centre – to remember and reclaim who you are.

Work with this book slowly and savour the process. You may want to read it all the way through once, and then come back to do the work. I would personally recommend that you work through the book chapter by chapter on your first time along the path, ideally spending at least a week, possibly a month, with each. After that, you can come back and revisit any chapters as and when you need to.

I have included a number of reclamation rituals throughout this book that are intended to help you to do the work to uncover the Goddess within. Take your time with these rituals; get to know the Goddess and yourself in a deep way as this is how you will make the most profound discoveries and changes in your life.

But the biggest reminder that I want to give you here, at the beginning of this journey together, is that the Goddess, the feminine, cannot be understood with the mind. The mind is masculine and the more we try to grasp and control the feminine and mould her into something that makes logical sense and can be put into a spreadsheet, the more she will elude us. The feminine is energy, a felt sense; she is body wisdom, intuition, deep inner knowing and the unseen.

It may sound a little mystical, but the feminine is not something you can necessarily explain in words; she is beyond words and so I ask that you *feel* the words I have written in this book rather than read and try to logically understand them. I ask you to see this as an energy transmission rather than a book, and that you read from your heart rather than your mind. I ask that you feel how the Goddess is showing up in your life and experience and embody it rather than trying to make sense of it.

This may be difficult to accept at first as you want to grasp and understand all of this, but the only way you will do that is to feel her, embody her, invite her in and, most of all, surrender to her. In doing so, your life will take on a whole new meaning and purpose and she will guide the way.

This journey isn't easy. In all honesty, the spiritual journey never is. It will challenge you, push you and help you to evolve and grow. It will bring forward all the lessons that your soul chooses to learn. But I promise you that it is so, so worth it.

As you reclaim the Goddess within and are reminded of who you are, before the world told you who to be, your life will never be the same again.

Welcome to the Goddess Path. If you're ready, let's begin . . .

Note: This is not a book just for women. Wherever you identify on the gender spectrum, we all have feminine, Goddess energy within us, just as we all have masculine energy within us. Anyone can walk the Goddess Path and use this journey to reclaim the divine Goddess within. I will use the word 'woman' in this book, as that is my lived experience and the truth from which I can speak. If this term does not resonate with you, please replace it with the one that does.

PART 1
THE DESCENT

The first part of our journey will help you look deep within so you can do the inner work needed to reclaim who you truly are. We'll descend into the underworld, unravelling, releasing and stripping away all that keeps you from being who you came here to be.

Before we do this, let's invoke the Goddess for her protection, guidance and strength as we begin this journey. You can use your own words or the ones below. Close your eyes, place your hands over your heart and ask the Goddess to be with you:

'Goddess, please surround me with your protection, love and guidance on this journey. Help me to be brave and courageous as I realise and release all that holds me back from my true Goddess self.'

Let's begin our journey along the Goddess Path's first six chapters with the descent.

'When you invoke and connect to the power of Shakti, and realise that you contain the divine feminine, the creative life force energy of the entire universe, you begin to see yourself and life differently.'

Chapter 1

RECLAIM THE GODDESS AND DIVINE FEMININE

Goddess energy is the essence of divine feminine energy. Sometimes known as Shakti, it is the creative life force energy that dances through the universe and brings everything to life. The earth, the heavens, the planets, the stars, all living beings and you are made of this primordial cosmic energy. When you connect to the Goddess, the Shakti energy within you, you gain access to a greater power source and higher levels of consciousness, and begin to experience yourself as part of something greater.

The wonderful news is that you are already a Goddess! This energy already moves through you, and you can access it at any time. You don't have to earn or fix or become worthy of your Goddess energy. Goddess energy is within every one of us. But somewhere along the way, you forgot, we forgot, the world forgot.

As a result of centuries of patriarchal rule, we live in a world that is heavily dominated by masculine energy and traits. We tend to celebrate doing, achieving, material success and profit, whereas the feminine qualities of intuition, inner wisdom, rest, receiving and flow are shunned and deemed useless or less worthy. This book is a call to awaken the long-forgotten, ignored, suppressed and denied feminine powers within each one of us. I truly believe that it was because of the immense power of the divine feminine that it was suppressed. There is nothing in the world more powerful than a woman who knows herself, trusts herself, believes in herself and is tapped into her feminine flow.

When you invoke and connect to the power of Shakti, and realise that you contain the divine feminine, the creative life force energy of the entire universe, you begin to see yourself and life differently. You take back your inner power, intuition, magic, knowing, worth, vision, purpose and full manifestation potential. You begin to realise who you truly are and what you're worth, and no longer accept less than you deserve. You connect to your sacred power, intuition and inner knowing, and begin to realise that you have within you the answer to every question and the solution to every problem. You stand strong in your authentic sense of self, making yourself and your wellbeing a priority, and you believe in yourself. You free the wild woman within and begin to care less about what society says as you allow yourself to become more untamed, paving your own way in the world and trusting where the Goddess energy wants to guide you. You claim your sensuality, passion and creative energy, and learn to understand and embrace your emotions and feelings. You begin to live in flow, honouring seasons and cycles. You see the magic and growth in everything, and you make your entire life a ritual and offering to the Goddess within, connecting you to a greater source of awareness.

Your soul came here to experience, learn and grow, and offer to the world what only you can offer – and it's the Goddess energy that will help you to bring to life the seeds of dreams, desires and purpose which are contained within you.

This is the guiding force of the universe which leads you along your soul path and helps you to experience all that your soul came here to experience and awaken all of who you came here to be. You are a Goddess.

One of the best ways to invoke the divine feminine energy is to work with Goddess and divine feminine archetypes, which help us to awaken their energy within ourselves.

Getting to Know the Goddess

A Goddess is a figure that represents the Shakti or the divine feminine in her many aspects. Each Goddess represents a unique expression of feminine energy that we can call upon to help us to awaken and embody the same within ourselves.

Some Goddesses are fierce, brave and powerful, while others are soft, gentle and nurturing, or passionate, sensual and wild. Each one holds gifts, qualities, traits and energies that we can call upon to share with us.

As we work with these Goddesses, their Shakti speaks to and awakens those parts of us that may have been dormant, hidden, suppressed or offline.

Each Goddess also comes with her own story or myth that helps connect us deeply to her, and we may find our own life stories told through theirs. We can then call upon the energy of the Goddess to help us to learn from her experience and lend us her knowledge, wisdom and strength.

We all have an inner Kali or Hecate, Artemis or Isis. We can consciously embody and call upon these Goddesses for support, depending on what we want to deepen into in our lives and ourselves.

In this book we'll meet different Goddesses in each chapter, whose energy and support you can call upon to deepen into the themes of that chapter. These are Goddesses who I have journeyed and worked with for many years, in many of the same ways I will share with you here. That way, I can speak from deep first-hand experience of the energies and wisdom these Goddesses have shared with me.

However, I want you to make this journey your own and experience the Goddess in your own unique way. There are hundreds and hundreds of Goddesses out there from many different cultures and religions that you can discover and work with who may resonate with you and your life journey more. Take some time to get clear on what you want the Goddess to help you with and then explore the Goddesses who most embody and exude what you are looking for.

As you journey through this book and get to know and work with these Goddesses, you will explore your perhaps yet unknown parts and bring them to life to understand yourself on a much deeper level.

When we start to recognise ourselves in these Goddesses, we begin to reclaim and embody the full expression of divine feminine energies. They will lend you their energy, their strength, their wisdom, their gifts and their voice until you can find your own. They will help you to reclaim the Goddess within.

As you walk the Goddess Path, some Goddesses will walk with you forever and others will come to you at the right time in the right way, just when you need them the most. Enjoy this journey of discovery, yet try to work with each Goddess for a length of time rather than short periods or trying to work with too many at once – like with any relationship, it will deepen the more time and energy you spend on it.

To help with this, I have tried to include the same Goddesses in various places throughout the book so that you can get to know them on a much more intimate level. For now, let me introduce you to some of the main divine feminine archetypes, with some ways to reclaim each one.

The Divine Feminine Archetypes

In the same way as the Goddesses, the divine feminine archetypes are universal feminine modes of expression which help you to tap into your powers and embody the highest expression of feminine energy. They are another way to connect to, or access, the feminine Goddess energies within.

Each of the archetypes holds different gifts, traits, power and wisdom which you can explore, tap into and awaken within you, helping you to grow into your full potential and access the fullness of feminine power.

It is likely that, over your lifetime, you have fallen into default modes of certain archetypes, which may mirror the different seasons in your life. For example, you may have spent many years as a mother. Or perhaps you've been living for some time in your queen energy building an empire. Or maybe you've been enjoying your carefree maiden season or working with your medicine woman archetype on a journey of healing and self-discovery.

But we are never just one archetype. As part of the Goddess Path, you want to be able to access, embrace, embody and experience them all and then be able to call upon whichever one is best needed for each season and situation in your life.

If you've been stuck in any one archetype for too long, you may find over time a little niggle of dissatisfaction creeping in. Or you may feel that you are in the shadow element of that archetype, burned out, exhausted or finding that what you have been doing for so long no longer brings you the pleasure or satisfaction that it once did. You may have loved your time as a mother, but, as your children grow older and begin to live their own lives, you may find a desire to know yourself outside of the parent role and do things for yourself once more. Or perhaps you've been hustling hard and built an incredible business or worked your way up the corporate ladder and now work doesn't bring you quite the joy it once did as there is a desire for more fun and play.

This is your invitation to spend more time with other archetypes to balance things out and allow other parts of you to take over for a little while. This will open a whole new world of energies for you to embody and explore, and, in turn, bring you a new lease of life. I have given you suggestions of which feminine archetypes you might embody and work with through each of the following chapters of the book and ways that you can do so.

Reclamation ritual

As you read through the list below, see which archetype(s) calls out to you as your most dominant and which ones you feel called towards to begin to work with or get to know more. Embody them for a day: how does she think, feel, act and move through the day? Get to know and awaken their energies within you.

The maiden

The maiden is free-spirited, youthful and playful. Sometimes known as the virgin, she is innocent, trusting, open-hearted and sees the good in everything and everyone. She moves through the world in a curious way, living in the moment and enjoying the journey. Call on the maiden when life has got too serious and you need to experience some joy, ease and fun.

Reclaim your inner maiden by:

○ Taking a day (or even an hour) off all responsibilities and to-do lists, and doing something that's purely for fun.

○ Inviting more play into your life. When was the last time you ran carefree into the sea or through a forest or laughed until you cried? How can you play more?

○ Spending a day seeing the good in everyone and everything, releasing any judgements and trusting that everyone is doing their best. Compliment everyone you meet on something good you see in them.

The mother

The mother offers unconditional love, and whether she has children of her own or not, she has a deep desire to nurture, care for and protect everyone around her, bringing out the best in them. She is a sense of home and belonging, the place we go to get nourished. Call on the mother when you need to be held and taken care of or when you need to fill your own cup enough to be able to give to others.

Reclaim your inner mother by:

○ Mothering yourself. Make it a habit to ask yourself regularly what you need – perhaps it's a quiet evening in to recharge, a couple of minutes in the morning to journal your feelings or a slow evening making a nourishing meal for yourself.

○ Caring for others, whether through cooking, cuddles or being a listening ear or supportive shoulder.

○ Connecting to Mother Earth and spending lots of time in nature. Let yourself be held by the great mother.

The warrioress

Also known as the huntress, the warrioress is a strong, fearless, independent woman on a mission. With a self-confident presence, she relies on no one but herself, lives life on her terms and fights for what she believes in (and for anyone else who can't fight for themselves). Call on the warrioress when you need to trailblaze your own path, get things done or need the courage to stand up for yourself.

Reclaim your inner warrioress by:

○ Challenging the status quo. Don't be afraid to ask questions, question authority and enter a healthy debate . . . it's the only way we'll ever make real change.
○ Spending time alone frequently, and during this time pleasing only yourself. Do things for you and only you.
○ Setting yourself regular goals and challenges, and going after them with your whole heart, believing in yourself.

The lover

Connected to her sensuality, sexuality, passion and pleasure, the lover radiates a magnetic, confident energy that makes her presence known. She loves deeply; herself, life and others, and desires meaningful and intimate relationships. She lives a life of bliss and turn-on. Call on the lover when you want to open yourself to fully experience pleasure, passion and aliveness, and to be present in and love your body.

Reclaim your inner lover by:

○ Enjoying a day of pure indulgence. Dress in beautiful clothes, eat all your favourite foods, enjoy a midday bath or massage, drink champagne for breakfast – whatever it is, indulge yourself.

○ Practising self-pleasure. Explore your body and the sensations, learn what you enjoy and use this time as sacred time dedicated purely to pleasure (with no need for an end result).

○ Writing yourself a love letter telling yourself everything you love most about yourself. Read the letter out loud to yourself often, especially in moments of low worth or doubt.

The healer

The healer takes our pain, suffering and grief, and shows us how to alchemise it into meaning and purpose. She is the midwife who supports us through childbirth or big life-changing transitions. She teaches us how to hold ourselves through our healing and, although she can't take it all away, she'll remain by your side through it all. Call on the healer when you're facing heartbreak, heartache or a big life change, or when you need to heal from anything past or present.

Reclaim your inner healer by:

○ Taking care of your body, mind, heart and soul. Do one thing daily for each to heal, hold and care for yourself and your wellbeing.

○ Investing in your own healing. This may be having therapy, practising forgiveness or apologising for ways in which you have hurt others.

○ Understanding that you can't heal or fix anyone else; you can support and encourage and hold, but you can't heal it for them.

The creatrix

A woman deeply connected to her feminine source of creative power, the creatrix is the vessel who brings things, whether children, hopes, dreams or ideas, to life. She weaves words, poems, energy, life, allowing whatever wants to come forth to be channelled through her in her own authentic self-expression. Call on the creatrix when you want to bring something to life, find your creativity or express yourself.

Reclaim your inner creatrix by:

○ Creating a new life story for yourself. If your world is filled with can'ts or fears or ways in which you hold yourself back, write a new story that empowers you.
○ Giving yourself time and space to just create. Paint, draw, dance, with no desired final result in sight – just allow creativity to flow through you.
○ Understanding that you get to create your own reality and bring whatever you want to life. Begin to believe in your feminine powers of creation.

The queen

A natural leader, the queen stands rooted in her own power, knowing who she is and what she wants. Devoted fully to herself and her life vision, she chooses where to place her precious energy, takes charge of her own destiny and lives a life of purpose and fulfilment. Call on the queen when you want to become the leader of your own life and embrace your power to live a life you truly want.

Reclaim your inner queen by:

○ Not settling for less. The queen knows what she is worth and is willing to wait to get it.

○ Investing in yourself. Whether that's courses, workshops, finding a coach or just completely backing yourself, do whatever you can to take you to your future vision of greatness.

○ Becoming your own authority. Although you do want to have a loyal team around you, stop outsourcing your life decisions and giving others power and control over your life.

The wise woman

Deeply connected to her inner wisdom, the wise woman trusts and follows her heart and soul. She has achieved self-mastery and her life is lived through following the magic of her inner knowings. Wise beyond her years, she is an old soul carrying the wisdom of her ancestors and elders. Call on the wise woman when you need answers and direction in life, and to trust your own intuition, inner wisdom and knowing.

Reclaim your inner wise woman by:

○ Cultivating your intuition and body wisdom. When you have any big decisions to make, drop out of your head and feel the answers in your body.

○ Sharing and teaching your wisdom. Know that, from your own lived life experience, you have wisdom to share that others need.

○ Carving out time for solitude and silence. The wise woman knows that all the answers you seek are found in silence.

The wild woman

Untameable, unknowable and uncontrollable, the wild woman is wild in every sense of the word. Unafraid of her depths and shadows, free of the shackles of society and fully in her authentic feminine power, she knows, owns and accepts all of herself. She is a force of nature calling you to be wild and free. Call on the wild woman when you have been censoring yourself and who you truly are, and want to break free to be all of you.

Reclaim your inner wild woman by:

○ Embracing and accepting all of yourself – from your big emotions to your shadows, your body, your opinions, your quirks, your uniqueness and everything in between. Love yourself fiercely.

○ Setting her free as much as you can. Put on your favourite song and dance, shake, crawl around on all fours, howl, stomp, sound and unleash the wild woman within.

○ Noticing when you censor yourself to be more likeable, palatable or agreeable, or when you dim to fit in or tame certain parts of you. Instead, begin to share more of your authentic truths.

The priestess

As a bridge between the physical and spiritual world, soul work, being of sacred service and following her purpose is the pathway of the priestess. Her world is one of rituals, ceremonies, miracles, magic and connection to spirituality, source and the divine. Her entire life is lived in devotion to a higher calling. Call on the priestess when you want to know and follow your purpose, commit to being of service and connect to your higher self and the divine.

Reclaim your inner priestess by:

○ Spending time daily in deep devotion such as meditating, journaling, praying, communing with nature or asking for help and guidance.
○ Inviting the divine into your life. Ask for and notice the signs, look for miracles, trust that you are being supported and guided, and see the divine in everything.
○ Being of more service. Even if you're not quite living the life you want just yet, think about how you can be of more service in your day-to-day life and use your gifts to support others.

The visionary

The visionary not only sees the future, she creates it. She has a clear vision of all that's possible, her fullest potential and what she wants to be expressed in the world through her. She weaves her own fate through her words, thoughts, actions and beliefs, and is a catalyst for change and transformation. Call on the visionary when you want to see the bigger picture of your life and the full potential of what's possible for you when you need to take action towards your future.

Reclaim your inner visionary by:

○ Connecting regularly to your future self; who is she, what is she doing, how does she act and move through the world, and how can you begin to embody more of her now, in the present?

- ⭘ Visualising daily what you want your future and life to be. See it all in as much detail as you can, then spend a few moments at the end receiving insights and guidance around how to get it.
- ⭘ Remembering that life is happening for you not to you. Everything happening is teaching you something and leading you somewhere.

The medicine woman

The shaman, the oracle, the witch, the sage, the wisdom keeper, the alchemist, she is connected to the true source of all healing, ancient magic, the earth, nature, our ancestors and cosmic energy. The medicine woman works in all realms to bring balance and healing, and carries and offers the medicine that we all need – the medicine for the soul. Call on the medicine woman when you know that you have healing gifts and talents, but are perhaps unsure of what they are or afraid to use them.

Reclaim your inner medicine woman by:

- ⭘ Sharing your medicine with the world, whether that is through your words, art, healing abilities, guidance, activism or intuitive wisdom. Know your medicine is needed in the world.
- ⭘ Connecting to and honouring the healing energies of the earth, nature, moon and planets, and worshipping the Goddess in these things.
- ⭘ Reconnecting to your ancestral lines and all the women who have come before you. Look at any healing that may need doing and wisdom and lessons that can be gained from your ancestors.

Invoking the Divine Feminine

Through this book, you will hear me speak often about invoking the Goddess and/or divine feminine archetypes, and so I wanted to make clear here what that means and how to do it.

The word 'invoke' means to call upon a deity or higher power for support, help, inspiration, blessings or assistance. As you invoke the Goddesses or feminine archetypes, you access the higher powers of the divine feminine and allow them to come through and support you in your life.

The feminine loves devotion, ritual and reverence, and the more you call upon the Goddess, the divine feminine, the more she will weave her magic through your life and help you to awaken to her energy.

We will look at daily rituals in Chapter 5, but, to begin with, feel the Goddess, talk to her, ask for her help and guidance, and feel how she shows up in your body and your life. Here are some ways you can start to invoke the Goddess as you begin your journey along the Goddess Path.

Create a Goddess altar

If you've come across any of my work before, you'll know that I am big on altars! An altar is a sacred space that you devote to your spiritual practices. It only needs to be a small space, ideally somewhere calm and quiet, and it's here that you will go to connect with the Goddess daily.

Make your altar beautiful, so that it represents the divine feminine. You may dress it with gorgeous cloths, flowers, crystals and candles. Add statues or a picture of the Goddess or archetype you are working with so that you can connect to her energies. Go to your altar each day to meditate, pray, journal or just to sit in silence with the Goddess and feel her energies.

△ *Say prayers to the Goddess* △

I know the word prayer can sometimes get lost in its more modern-day meaning, but I pray to the Goddess daily.

To me, prayer is you talking to the Goddess, invoking the higher power of the feminine and asking for her help and support in any areas you may need it. So often we struggle with things, when all we need to do is give it up to something greater to allow the answers, clarity and guidance to come through.

Get in the habit of saying daily prayers – either written down in a journal or spoken out loud – to the Goddess, thanking her for showing up in your life and asking her to weave her energy through you to awaken the Goddess and divine feminine within. Ask her to work through you and to help you to see, hear and know what you need to see, hear and know.

If you need more strength, courage, wisdom, insight, sensuality, flow, softness or trust, ask her to help you to awaken these things within you so that you may connect more deeply to the full feminine force.

△ *Use Goddess affirmations* △

Affirmations are positive phrases that are repeated to help you to overcome self-sabotage, limiting beliefs and unhelpful thoughts and behaviours. Over time, they encourage self-belief and inner confidence, and help you to begin to embody who and what you want to become.

When we say Goddess affirmations, they help to ignite and activate the feminine power within. They begin to remind you that you are a Goddess, and you are capable of anything that you set your mind, heart and soul to.

Your words are like spells – they hold such immense power, so begin to use them wisely. Imagine that you are literally casting a spell with the words you speak – what are you speaking into being? Become more intentional with your words and use them to reclaim your inner Goddess.

I'll offer specific affirmations at the end of each chapter, but some you may want to begin with are:

○ 'I am a Goddess.'
○ 'I honour the Goddess.'
○ 'I allow divine feminine energy to flow through me.'
○ 'My inner Goddess guides me.'
○ 'I trust the ancient wisdom and guidance of the Goddess.'

△ *Journal to the Goddess* △

You may want to get yourself a beautiful journal at the beginning of your journey along the Goddess Path that you can dedicate to the Goddess. In this, journal to the Goddess, asking for her wisdom and guidance, and baring your heart and soul to her.

You may also write a question to the Goddess, then pause, take a few deep breaths, feel her energy come close and then write yourself an answer from the Goddess. Journal too on the ways in which the Goddess is showing up in your life, how you are changing and growing through this journey, and your realisations, breakthroughs and insights along the way.

Harness Goddess crystal magic

If you want to feel the Goddess with you at all times, set intentions on a crystal that you can keep on your altar, meditate with or carry around with you as a touchstone to remind you that she is always with you. Here are some of the best crystals to harness Goddess energy:

○ **Moonstone:** holding the feminine energy of the moon, moonstone will help you to channel lunar energy to connect with your emotions, intuition and inner Goddess. It will help you to link to your own natural rhythms and cycles, and trust in yourself and your inner wisdom.

○ **Rose quartz:** the crystal of unconditional love, rose quartz is the embodiment of feminine energy helping you to know, love and care for yourself as the Goddess that you are. It will help you to know your value and worth, and heal and open your heart.

○ **Selenite:** named after Selene, Goddess of the moon, selenite will help to clear and cleanse your energy so that you can connect to your inner Goddess more easily. It also links you to your soul's purpose, which the Goddess wants to bring to life through you.

○ **Labradorite:** a crystal of magic, intuition and protection, labradorite will remind you of your inner power and awaken you to your inner knowing. It will help you to find courage and creativity, and connect to your third eye chakra (we'll meet this in Chapter 6) to see the truth.

○ **Chrysocolla:** often called the Goddess or wise woman crystal, chrysocolla teaches us how to reclaim our divine feminine and Goddess energies, wisdom and gifts, and begin to share them with the world around us.

I hope that through this chapter you have started to get to know the Goddess at a deeper level and how she shows up and weaves her way through your life. Let's look now at how you can call upon her to help you to reclaim your self-worth, one of the most important foundations for reclaiming the Goddess within.

'One of the most powerful forces in the world is a woman who knows her worth.'

Chapter 2

RECLAIM YOUR SELF-WORTH

The next stop along the Goddess Path is realising your self-worth, as this is one of the main foundations of embracing your inner Goddess.

Self-worth is the inner sense and belief that you are enough. Having a sense of high self-worth means that you value yourself and know that you are worthy and deserving of being treated well and having all that you desire in life. Everything in your life and your thoughts, feelings, behaviours, actions and choices are dependent on how worthy and deserving you feel within yourself. If you don't feel worthy of being treated well, you are more likely to stay in unhealthy jobs, relationships and situations, not believing there is anything better out there for you. You will accept less from life, shrink yourself, downplay your abilities and what you have to offer the world, suppress what you truly want and always settle for less than you deserve, which further compounds your beliefs that you are not worthy of any better.

When you doubt yourself and your abilities, you will find it hard to believe in yourself, and this will hold you back from going after what you truly want in life. You will never be able to create the life that you want or have what you truly desire if you don't believe that you're worthy of it. For example, you're unlikely to apply for your dream job if you don't believe, deep down, that you have what it takes to be able to fulfil the role. You may desire a deep meaningful relationship, but, unless you believe yourself to be worthy of that depth of love, you will never be able to receive it and will instead sabotage your chances of true love. Your ability to create, manifest and go after what you want in life depends on how much you believe you are deserving of having it. This keeps you in an endless spiral of wanting more for yourself and perhaps deep down knowing that you deserve better, but not quite being able to break free and get it.

When you are not safe and secure in yourself, with a strong sense of your values, worth and your inner Goddess, you are more likely to abandon yourself. This is why we very often look for our sense of self-worth in the outside world – in this day and age, predominantly on social media waiting for 'likes' to roll in. We seek approval and validation from others and base our worth on our achievements, job, relationships and appearance, believing that we have to somehow earn our place in the world. We give all of our power away to external sources, which we allow to decide our worth for us.

We also tend to allow a big part of our identity to be wrapped up in the externals. When we initially meet someone, the first things we tend to tell them about who we are is where we live, the job we do, the partner we have, the car we drive, who we know, the things we have, what we've achieved – all very valuable information, but none of this refers to who you actually are.

Our sense of self-worth is further eroded by the world of advertising, which is constantly telling us that we need something outside us to feel worthy – you'll finally be happy when you have that body, this mascara, that holiday, this outfit, this face cream . . . the list goes on. And it never ends. We live in a consumer culture that profits from us always feeling like we are never quite enough, and women in particular have been pitted against each other for decades, putting our bodies, behaviours and beauty standards up for opinion, judgement and debate. From a very young age, you have been subliminally told that there is something wrong with you and the way that you are, but it's time to break that spell.

The truth is that your worth and your value do not need to be earned in the world; they just need to be remembered and reclaimed. It's time to remember who you truly are, before the world told you who to be.

You are more than enough just as you are. And when you remember this, you become unstoppable. You will begin to know yourself, understand yourself, accept yourself, value yourself and love yourself. You will begin to show up in the fullest, most authentic presence of you and allow the Goddess that you are to be fully seen and shine. You will start to trust yourself and believe in yourself, and this enables you to begin to reach for all that you are truly worthy of in life.

One of the most powerful forces in the world is a woman who knows her worth. You get to decide your worth, and it begins here.

Give Yourself What You're Seeking

When your sense of self-worth is dependent on anything outside of you it can always be taken away, which is why it's so important that you claim it for yourself. Imagine that I click my fingers and everything external is suddenly taken away from you (your material possessions, status, job/career, relationships, friendships, achievements, accomplishments, and so on). How would that make you feel? Would your sense of self-worth and identity disappear with all of these external things? Who would you be without them?

The first thing you need to realise is that you are not your age, your social media following, your to-do list, your dress size, your job, your achievements, your bank balance or your relationship status, and none of these things define your worth – unless you allow them to. It may be worth taking some time here to reflect on where you look outside of yourself for approval and validation, and what you depend on to give you a sense of worth.

Ask yourself, who do you seek the most approval from in your life? Do you look for validation in the number of likes you get on social media, or in your accomplishments, or in the attention you get from others? Do you worry too much about what others think of you and allow that to hold you back from doing certain things? Are you nobody if you're not in a relationship, or only feel like somebody because of the job that you do, or friendship circles you move in?

Pause here in this moment to really reflect on these questions and what comes up for you. Perhaps take a little longer here to journal on this before you move on. The answers to these questions will give you such powerful insight into where you outsource your value and worth, and where you need to claim it back. This begins with knowing and understanding yourself and giving yourself what you seek from others and anything outside of yourself.

Dig deep and try to identify what it is that you are seeking from these things. If it's approval, start to approve of yourself; if you're looking to be chosen, start to choose yourself; if you want permission to be who you are and do what you want to do, give yourself permission; if you want praise, start to praise yourself.

You also teach others how to treat you so, if you want other people to understand you, you have to first understand yourself. If you want others to love you, you have to first love yourself. If you want others to respect you and treat you well, you have to first respect and treat yourself well.

It all starts with you, and the more you can give yourself what you are looking for, the less you'll need to seek it from anything or anyone outside you, and the more you'll realise you're worthy and deserving just by being you.

By the end of this book, I want you to be able to tell me who you are. I want you to be able to tell me of your greatness, your worth and your purpose. I want you to be able to tell me of your values, your hopes and dreams and desires, your wildness, your shadows, what you're good at, what makes you happy, what you can bring to the world and everything that makes up the very essence of you.

Reclamation ritual

Once a month, or even once a fortnight, take yourself out on a date. If the thought of going somewhere alone terrifies you, I encourage you even more so to do this. If you can't spend a few hours or even a day with you, how can you expect anyone else to want to?

Spending time with yourself means that you get to know yourself, what you like and how truly wonderful you really are to be around. It means that you learn to self-source what you need and spend time really getting to know yourself.

Personally, I believe that every Goddess should travel on her own at least once in her life – you will learn all you need to know about yourself. For me, travelling to India alone was one of the most life-changing things I ever did. I had to be there for myself, trust myself and make decisions for myself. In times of loneliness, fear or uncertainty, I used to place my cheek against my own shoulder, put my arms around myself and say, 'Don't worry Kirst, I'm here, I've got you and I'll take care of you.' I learned so much about myself through those months and developed such a deep trust and love for myself that it was worth every hard moment. I learned that you can never be lonely when you like who you're alone with.

Travelling may be a stretch to begin with, but start with an hour, then half a day, maybe even a night and build up as you go. I promise, once you realise what great company you are and how fabulous you are to hang out with, you'll never be in as much doubt about your worth again.

Make Friends with Your Inner Critic

Start noticing how you speak to yourself, as this is a good indication of your current levels of self-worth and how you allow others to talk to you and treat you.

When you make a mistake, what is the first thing you tell yourself? Is it how useless you are and how you can't do anything right? Or do you support yourself, understanding that you made a mistake and can learn from this and do better next time? The lower your levels of self-worth, the louder your inner critic tends to be.

Your inner critic is the nagging inner voice that judges, criticises, compares and questions everything, and tells you all the ways you're not good enough. It is shaped by your previous life experiences and, in its own way, is trying to protect you and help you to avoid what it sees as mistakes and failures. I can hazard a good guess, though, that, if you heard someone speak to your best friend the way you sometimes speak to yourself, you'd jump in and say, 'Hold on a minute, don't talk to her like that!'

Reclaiming your inner narrative is an important part of reclaiming your self-worth, and so begin to gently challenge that little voice within, and turn your inner voice into one that supports and encourages you. A powerful way to do this is to simply ask, 'Is that true?' So when your inner critic is telling you that you can't do anything right or that you're not good enough, ask yourself 'Is that true?'

There are times when we can use the voice of the inner critic to help us to learn and grow and realise where we can do better, but chances are a lot of what the voice is telling you isn't true at all.

Deep down, your Goddess within knows that you are a good person and doing your best, and the more you can realise and recognise that, the more you can encourage and support yourself. So, begin a dialogue with the critic and flip the script. If the critic whispers, 'Why would they give you the job?', ask the critic, 'Why wouldn't they give me the job? I'm hard-working, smart and have so much to offer to the position, they'd be lucky to have me.' When the critic says, 'Why would they like/love you?', ask, 'Why wouldn't they like/love me? I'm beautiful, kind, loyal, fun to be around, a good listener and make a really good friend/lover/partner/colleague.'

Start to reinforce to yourself all the reasons why you are enough and do deserve the best. Tell yourself often that you are doing your best, praise yourself each time you do something well, talk to yourself in the way that you would want your best friend or lover to talk to you, and watch your inner narrative and levels of self-worth begin to change.

Reclamation ritual

Each morning, look in the mirror, gaze at yourself and smile. Notice if the inner critic stirs and, instead of listening to that voice, compliment yourself on something. Find something to love about yourself in that moment and celebrate the Goddess that you are. Take this supportive, loving energy with you into the day ahead.

At the end of each day, return to the mirror and tell yourself everything you did well today and what you are proud of yourself for. Notice if any judgement stirs around you celebrating yourself or if you're unable to accept these compliments.

Learn to celebrate yourself all through the day – each time you do something brave or make a good decision or show up for yourself, congratulate and praise yourself. You are so worthy of celebration and recognition, and your Goddess will begin to shine through so much more when you recognise her in all of her glory.

Choose You

Choosing you is one of the most powerful things that you can do to reclaim your sense of self-worth.

Recently, a dear friend of mine was ghosted and went into a spiral of 'what's wrong with me, what did I do wrong, why am I not good enough' – a dialogue that I'm sure is familiar to so many of us. Witnessing this, it really hit home how we put so much of our value and worth in being chosen by others, believing that someone else choosing us makes us somehow accepted and worthy. She is a wonderful, smart, intelligent, beautiful Goddess and here she was allowing the fact that someone else didn't choose her to make her doubt her worth and entire existence.

It's in times like these that we get to choose ourselves. As much as they hurt at the time, these moments are such powerful teachers and shine a light on where we don't truly feel worthy and where we still give our power away and seek approval and validation from outside of ourselves.

When you get rejected, whether in a relationship or job, does your sense of self-worth and value go with it? How often do you go on a date and spend the whole time worrying about whether they like you, without ever stopping to consider whether you actually like them?

Choosing you means beginning to show up for yourself, especially in the hard and challenging moments of life. It means that you give yourself the support, love, care, attention and approval that you are seeking from others. It means knowing that you are worthy, deserving and enough, even when others can't or don't want to choose you.

So often when we are in a spiral because someone hasn't messaged back, or we feel rejected or abandoned, we lose ourselves even more by going into all the reasons why there is something wrong with us or how we aren't loveable or good enough to make someone else want to stay. This causes us to further reject and abandon ourselves, making us feel even less worthy. What if, in those moments, you chose yourself? What if you looked yourself in the eyes in the mirror and told yourself, 'I choose you. It doesn't matter whether they choose you, because I choose you'? Try it next time you are in a self-worth spiral – it's one of the most powerful things you will ever do for yourself.

Then pause to get really honest about how you are feeling in that moment. It may be that you feel rejected, unworthy of ever truly being loved or never chosen. Notice the story that you are telling yourself about what this rejection means about you. This gives you a beautiful insight into the unhealed parts of you, the parts that still seek validation, approval, love and acceptance from something or someone outside you.

Imagine if the friend I mentioned earlier had been truly rooted in her sense of self-worth and knew without doubt that she was a good person deserving of the best. That's not to say the ghosting wouldn't have been hurtful or confusing initially, but rather that she wouldn't have taken it personally or made it mean anything about her or her worthiness. She would have understood that he was likely going through something in his life and that the ghosting said way more about him than it did about her. She would have held herself in the initial moments of upset and recognised the parts of her that felt abandoned, let down, not chosen or whatever her internal story was – and she would have held and chosen these parts, giving herself exactly what she needed in that moment.

Furthermore, from doing this and valuing herself, she would know that she deserved better than this kind of behaviour and that this wasn't the kind of person or relationship she wants or even has time for in her life. She would have chosen herself over putting up with bad behaviour to be chosen by someone else.

When you choose yourself, it means that you don't need anyone else to choose you. Each time you choose you, you empower yourself, reclaim your self-worth, affirm how deserving you are of the best in life and allow the Goddess within you to begin to rise.

Reclamation ritual

Much of your worth is based on the stories you tell yourself about who you are and what you are worthy of. Whenever you notice yourself in a self-doubt spiral, feeling rejected or abandoned, or looking for something outside you, journal on what story you are telling yourself.

It may be a story of 'I am never chosen', or 'This always happens to me', or 'I'm not pretty, sexy or young enough.' Notice if you're the victim in the story, waiting to be chosen or for something or someone outside of you to fix you. See if you can trace back to where this story came from, whether that was something from your childhood or something the outside world told you. Notice how many other times in your life you have told yourself this same story.

Now, begin to tell yourself a new story. One where you are a Goddess, and you are beautiful, bold, brave and magnificent. A story in which you are more than enough and know your true power and worth. A story where you are worthy and deserving of the best. A story where you know that you have everything you need already within you.

You can begin to tell yourself a new story anytime you choose.

INVOKE THE GODDESS

As we begin this journey together, I want to introduce you to one of my all-time favourite Goddesses, **Durga**.

Durga has been on my team for well over a decade, and I can honestly say that invoking and embodying her energy has been life-changing for me. When teaching a yoga retreat in France many years ago, I told the story of Durga and we dedicated practices and offerings to her, inviting her energy into our lives. Our mantra became 'WWDD?' – 'What would Durga do?' – and, over the course of that retreat, and for many years after, in moments where we doubted ourselves or our abilities or our worth, we'd ask ourselves 'WWDD?', and allow her essence to awaken within us and bring us strength, courage and power.

Durga is a Hindu Goddess known for providing protection, strength and helping you to access the true source of your inner power and knowing. She is a warrior Goddess; fierce, primal, wild, untamed, often called upon to battle with dark forces. She is kundalini energy, a form of divine feminine energy which is the primal force behind spiritual awakenings and lies like a coiled serpent at the base of your spine. Yet she has a motherly energy that holds you tenderly and gently as she pushes you towards your full potential and all that she knows you are capable of.

If you've ever woken up in the middle of the night knowing that you just can't keep living the life you are living, you've already met Durga. Durga calls you home; back to yourself, your soul, your power, your dreams. She is the Goddess to call upon when you know that things in your life need to change, but you can't seem to find the strength to do it. Or when you are facing challenges and find yourself afraid, doubting and stuck in your fears and can't see a way out. Or when you're in a self-doubt spiral and can't find the belief in yourself.

Calling upon Durga in your life always comes with a gentle warning. Once you invite her in, it's likely that she will initially turn your life upside down as she propels you into what you need for your highest good. She will remove what is in the way, drive you to take action and show you where you are settling for less, asking you to face up to where you are staying small and allowing doubts and fears to hold you back.

Bringing a warrior-like strength, she will push you to transform, evolve, come out of your comfort zone, confront your fears, face obstacles and problems head on, know your worth and value, and embrace the fullness of who you are. She will become your greatest supporter, your protector, your guardian, lending you her courage when you feel afraid and helping you to awaken your own inner warrior to fight for, stand up for and speak up for yourself.

When you invite Durga into your life, she will help you to get to know your own needs and be fearless in expressing them, and to find an unshakeable belief in yourself and all that you are worthy of. If you're truly ready to know your worth and step into your fullest power, presence and potential, it's time to meet Durga for yourself.

Create a Durga altar

○ Create a sacred space where you can go to daily to worship and connect to Durga's energy. This may contain images or symbols of Durga or anything that represents her strength, courage and wisdom. Her colours are red, yellow, gold and orange, so incorporate these, and perhaps include a candle you can light daily to welcome in Durga's energy.

○ Sit with your altar daily, saying prayers to Durga for anywhere you need her support, guidance and strength.

Meditate with Durga

Meet Durga in your meditation. You may imagine her strength and power in your body or visualise her sitting with you sharing her wisdom and giving you strength and empowerment. Commit to sitting with Durga's energy for 5–10 minutes a day every day for 30 days and see what changes begin to take place within you.

Use Durga's mantra

Durga's mantra is *Om Dum Durgayei Namaha*. This is a prayer honouring her. Repeated silently as a form of mantra meditation or out loud to harness the vibration of the words, this mantra will invoke Durga's energy and protection. Mantras are traditionally repeated 108 times, a number that's said to bring you into harmony with the universe and your higher spiritual self. Try chanting Durga's mantra daily (you can get mala beads to help you with the counting or there is a guided chant on my website) and watch your life transform.

Call upon Durga

At the beginning of each day or in moments of struggle, doubt or fear, simply ask Durga to be there with you. Tell her what you need help with and ask for her protection, support and guidance. Notice where you feel her energy in your body. Is it in your belly or heart? What does it feel like? Is it like an almighty roar or a gentle nudge forward, or does she wrap herself around you like a protective cloak? The more you connect to Durga, the more you'll feel her energy flow through you, guiding you forwards.

Ask 'What would Durga do?'

When you're uncertain, unsure or when you need some extra courage to make a big decision, ask yourself 'WWDD?' Let the energy of the Goddess guide you, and embody her boldness, bravery and fearlessness to help you to step into your own power and courage.

Embody the Archetypes

The queen

Call upon your inner queen to show you that you are worthy and deserving of all that you desire. Spend a day or two in your queen energy feeling into how you would act, what you would ask for and what you would/wouldn't put up with if you were living as the queen you truly are.

The warrioress

Call upon your inner warrioress when you need to show up for yourself, stand up for yourself or speak up for yourself. Feel her energy supporting you, fighting for you and reminding you of who you are.

Stand in Your Self-Worth

Start to stand tall and take up the space you deserve in the world. At the beginning of each day, right before you walk into a room or in moments when you are doubting yourself and your worth, stand tall.

Plant your feet on the earth, lengthen through the crown of your head, draw your shoulders back and down, hold your head up high, open your heart wide and feel your inner Goddess filling your entire being.

AFFIRMATIONS TO RECLAIM YOUR SELF-WORTH

- ○ 'I am worthy and deserving of all that I desire.'
- ○ 'I am enough, just as I am.'
- ○ 'I love and approve of myself.'
- ○ 'I deserve happiness (or love, abundance, joy or anything else).'
- ○ 'I am at peace with my past.'
- ○ 'I am my own best friend.'
- ○ 'I am unique; there is no one else like me.'

You have started to reclaim your value and worth and know that you are enough just as you are, as the Goddess intended you to be. Taking these new levels of self-worth with us, let's use these now to begin to create some boundaries.

'Boundaries are one of the greatest acts of self-love. They help you to protect yourself, honour yourself and value yourself as the Goddess that you are.'

Chapter 3

RECLAIM YOUR BOUNDARIES

We continue our journey along the Goddess Path with the reclamation of your boundaries.

Boundaries are one of the greatest acts of self-love. They create more self-worth, self-trust and self-respect. They teach others about ways in which you want to be treated. They help you to protect yourself, honour yourself and value yourself as the Goddess that you are. Without strong boundaries, we can end up people-pleasing, saying yes when we mean no, and no when we mean yes, and constantly abandoning ourselves with no real sense of who we are or what we want, need and desire.

The more we do this, the more we build an inner sense of resentment and anger around constantly doing things that we don't want to do. We end up feeling like we never get our needs met or that people are always taking advantage of us, and no one understands or cares about us. This can lead to burnout, isolation and even more people-pleasing and self-abandon as we try to get our needs met, yet each time we self-abandon we lose trust in ourselves, our boundaries become weaker and it becomes a vicious circle.

If you take on other people's moods, often feel guilty for no apparent reason, struggle to say no or ask for what you need, often feel criticised or misunderstood or somehow responsible for everyone else and their feelings, the chances are that you could benefit from setting some boundaries. Take some time now to consider where you are not nurturing, claiming and listening to the Goddess within because you are too busy worrying about what everyone else needs. The more you ignore the Shakti within you, the more you'll disconnect from yourself and your feminine energy. Yes, the feminine is nurturing, nourishing and caretaking, but not at the expense of yourself. The first person you need to nurture, nourish and take care of is YOU.

When you create healthy boundaries, they draw an invisible line around you that separates you from others. For any of you old enough to remember the legendary film *Dirty Dancing*, it's like that scene – 'This is my dance space, this is yours.' A boundary says, 'This is my physical and energetic space, and my needs, feelings and responsibilities, and these are yours.' It helps you to know where you end and others begin, and what you are and aren't responsible for.

Healthy boundaries help us to realise that it's not our job to fix, save or rescue others, and that we are not responsible for other people's feelings, emotions, decisions, happiness or lives. Boundaries begin to foster self-trust as, through setting and maintaining boundaries, you begin to feel safe with yourself, knowing that you will look after you and not abandon you for the sake of others. They also help others to feel safe around you as they know where they are with you, what you want and need, and what is expected, acceptable and allowed.

You may have heard the saying that expectations are the biggest killers of relationships. Boundaries help us to set realistic expectations with ourselves and others, and to communicate and ask for what we want rather than just expecting something.

We can often fear that setting boundaries will push people away, yet the truth is that they foster more safety and connection as there is no longer any underlying resentment, disappointment, frustration, confusion or doubt. Boundaries are not there to keep people out, they are there to protect you and honour your needs, helping you to care for yourself and let others know what you will and won't accept and how you want to be treated.

When you first begin to set boundaries, it can be extremely challenging, especially if you've spent most of your life having none. But you will need strong boundaries as you walk the Goddess Path. As you begin to explore, discover and free more of yourself and start to change, there will be a push back from those around who want you to stay the same, and this may cause you to want to collapse your boundaries and people-please even more. Your transformation very often highlights where they need to change, but they are not brave enough. It is often easier for them to try to shame you into staying the same rather than looking at their own lives. In these moments, it's so important to remember that the only people who will resist or have an issue with your boundaries are those who benefited from you not having any.

It is also natural and normal for people to fall away as you no longer have the same things in common or share the same values. As sad as this can be, trust the process – it creates the space for other people to come in who are more aligned with who you are becoming.

Hold true to you, embody more of your inner Goddess and know that you walking this path is an inspiration to so many other women out there. The more and more we stand in our Goddess power and claim our own boundaries, the more we encourage and accept others doing the same.

Types of Boundaries

There are many types of boundaries, but here are a few that you may want to consider at the beginning of your boundary journey.

Physical boundaries

These include your personal space, taking care of your body, how you're comfortable being touched/hugged, self-care, when and what you eat and drink, and downtime and rest.

You may not wish to have people pushing you to drink on a night out, for example, or encouraging you to be active when you want to rest and relax. There may be certain people or situations in which you're not comfortable being hugged or times you wish to prioritise exercise for your wellbeing.

Emotional boundaries

These include what you are comfortable sharing with others, what you are comfortable them sharing with you and how much you're available to support others.

This may mean asking for time and space when you need it or being honest when you don't have the emotional capacity to deal with someone else's problems at that time. It may mean asking for someone not to discuss certain topics with you or not making yourself responsible for how others are feeling and trying to fix them.

Time/resource boundaries

These include how, where and with whom you choose to spend your time, money and energy. These are precious commodities, and these boundaries ensure that you spend them wisely. Perhaps you need to set a boundary with the friend who is always late that you'll only wait 15 minutes in the future, or that you only have 10 minutes available to chat to the person who calls you for hours at a time or in the middle of a working day. It may be turning down an expensive spa day right before pay day or the invite of a night out when you are depleted or exhausted.

Reclamation ritual

Now that you know a bit more about boundaries, what is the most important boundary that you need to set for yourself right now? Or in what life area or with whom do you most need to create a boundary?

○ Commit to setting and maintaining one boundary this week. First, get clear on why you are setting this boundary, so that you can remind yourself of this in the moments when you want to collapse your boundary. For example, it may be that you are setting a boundary not to discuss a certain topic with your family to take care of your emotional or mental health, or that you will say 'no' to the friend who wants to come over every night so that you can take an evening for yourself to rest and self-care.

○ Next, you may practise how you are going to set the boundary and what you will say. When we first begin, we can tend to set hard boundaries where we initially go too hard or push people away, but you will get better the more you practice. Speak from your heart and be clear and concise about your boundary and what your needs are. Remember to speak from 'I' and try not to blame or make it about the other person – this is about you setting a boundary for *you*.

Get to Know Who You Are

To have strong boundaries you need a deep sense of self-identity and knowing who you are and what you value and want. It's this sense of the truth of yourself that you build boundaries around.

To do this, it really helps to identify your core values, as they enable you to know and understand yourself and what is important to you. This means you can live a more authentic and purposeful life as your values inform your decisions, behaviours and choices, and allow you to create boundaries around who you are and what matters to you most.

Once you know your values, you'll notice that it's when you're living out of alignment with them that you feel the most lost, uncertain, stuck, unhappy and powerless, and this guides you as to where boundaries are needed in your life. Remember too that your values can and will change as you evolve and grow, so spend regular time in self-reflection and checking in with what is important for you.

Reclamation ritual

○ Identify your top five values. There are lots of lists of values online that you can search for. Begin by getting rid of any that don't resonate with you at all. Try to narrow down to your top ten, then your top five.

○ Once you know your values, begin to get honest about where in your life you are not living in alignment with these values. These will likely be the places where your life feels sticky or unfulfilling, and where you are most likely not honouring your boundaries.

○ Use your values as a guiding force for your boundaries. For example, if one of your main values is peace, you may create boundaries around how much time you spend with people who bring chaos into your life, or putting yourself in social environments that make you feel anxious. If you value truth, you may create boundaries around others wanting to gossip with you or getting involved in any 'he said, she said' situations, preferring to go directly to the source for answers.

Explore Your Boundary Beliefs

It's time for a deep dark confession from me, but I feel we know each other well enough now for that. Ready? I used to say yes to so many invites, knowing full well that I didn't want to and wouldn't go and would make an excuse nearer the time/on the day (sorry to anyone I did this to).

The more I got to know myself, the ickier this felt as it was so out of alignment with who I wanted to be and how I wanted to show up in full authenticity. I'd feel terrible cancelling and would sometimes not let people know at all and just not show up. Horrible behaviour.

It's only when I really sat with this truth that I uncovered a deeply held belief that people wouldn't like me if I didn't say yes, and they would never invite me again. Yet, after me letting them down, the likelihood was that they wouldn't, and it became a self-fulfilling prophecy. So, to try to get people to like me, I'd say yes even more, and on and on the cycle continued.

Rather than me pushing through that uncomfortable moment of saying, 'No thank you', which would have maintained the relationship and fostered trust, respect and intimacy, I behaved in a way that likely created the same outcome I was trying to avoid in the first place. That's what lack of boundaries does for us.

We often collapse our boundaries, especially as women, as we want to be seen as the 'good girl' or 'nice girl' or play the role of taking care of everyone else because we've been taught it's selfish to put ourselves first and so we please others at the expense of ourselves. Or we may be spiritually bypassing, using our spirituality to avoid facing issues or uncomfortable situations and making it all 'love and light' or excusing other people's behaviours. Over time, though, this causes self-abandon and inner resentment.

Reclamation ritual

○ Take some time to recognise the fears you have around creating boundaries. Dig deep, get honest and vulnerable. What deep belief has held you back from creating boundaries in the past?

○ Once you have identified it, you can use this to help you create future boundaries. For example, 'If I wasn't afraid that they wouldn't like me, what would I do?'

Reclaim Your Sacred No

Reclaiming the word 'no' is one of the first stages in setting boundaries, yet, for a little word, it's hard for so many of us to say. Because it's so hard to say, we tend to make excuses, over explain and try to justify why we don't want to do something, which further makes us feel like we are doing something wrong.

I remember how hard it was when I did first start to say no to invites. I'd give all the reasons why I couldn't go and talk round in circles with six-minute voice notes all about how 'I'd love to, but . . .' Each time I did this, it left me feeling so guilty, and when I dug deeper into this, it's because I was abandoning myself and my needs and making myself feel like I was somehow letting someone down or doing something wrong. But over time I realised that me saying no to them was me saying yes to me and, ever since that realisation, I've started to say yes to me so much more.

Start practising no as a complete sentence in itself (you may add thank you after it if that makes you feel better!) without feeling the need to make excuses for yourself. Remember, too, that anything before a 'but' is bul**hit. We often make excuses of 'I'd love to, but . . .' You wouldn't love to, or you'd do it. This is another way we make excuses for ourselves and our decisions, and it takes away our power.

Try instead: 'I would love to see you; this weekend is busy for me so how about next Wednesday?' or 'That sounds great, it's just not something I want to commit to right now. Let me get back to you.' Take back the power of your words and choices.

Reclamation ritual

Saying no can be uncomfortable, really uncomfortable. And so, your ritual is to sit in the discomfort of your no. The more you do this, the more you'll widen your window of tolerance. It's like an ice bath – the first time you go in, you may last 15 seconds and want to get out. The second time you might last 30 seconds, then 1 minute, then 3.

The first time you set a boundary your 'good girl' may jump in and say, 'actually, yes I will,' or your mind will tell you all the reasons the other person won't like you anymore or what a horrible person you are. But as you learn to sit in this discomfort, the easier it will become. In these moments, turn back to yourself, be there for yourself, soothe and encourage yourself, love and care for yourself. Remind yourself of why you set the boundary and that you have the right to make decisions that are best for you.

As you start to say no to things that no longer light you up, things that no longer serve you and things that no longer bring you joy, the more space you will create to say yes to all the things you want to do. Reclaiming your no helps you to also reclaim your yes. As Glennon Doyle says in her book *Untamed*, 'Every time you're given a choice between disappointing someone else and disappointing yourself, your duty is to disappoint that someone else. Your job throughout your entire life, is to disappoint as many people as it takes to avoid disappointing yourself.'

If you really struggle to initially say no, feel the Goddess within you. Feel her energy, power and strength fill you all the way up and allow her to lend you her voice and speak through you – 'no'.

Listen to Your Body Wisdom

As we learned in the Introduction, Goddess energy lives within our bodies, and when we begin to tune back into the innate wisdom of our bodies, we realise that they are always trying to communicate with us and show us something.

Your feelings are a powerful indicator of where your boundaries have been crossed, especially anger and resentment, which show up when you feel taken advantage of or don't feel appreciated. Alongside feeling discomfort, anxiety, fear, burnout, exhaustion or stress, you may also notice physical signs, such as your jaw tightening when someone is overstepping a boundary in a conversation or your heart clenching, stomach flipping or chest tightening. This is your body and inner Goddess energy trying to signal to you that something is not ok.

You can also turn to your body wisdom to help you to make decisions and set boundaries. Say you have received an invite to go somewhere and you're not sure whether to go. Close your eyes, take a few long, slow, deep breaths, and pay attention to your body. Then imagine saying yes and see what happens in your body. Imagine saying no and see what happens in your body. It may be that when you imagined saying yes, you felt your stomach clench, your heartbeat increase and your throat tighten. And when you imagined saying no, you felt a warmth within, a peace and stillness. This gives you your answer.

Reclamation ritual

This week, turn to your body wisdom for answers and guidance. Something I try to live by is that if it's not a full-body yes, it's a no. When I need to make a decision about doing something, I imagine saying yes, going and doing the thing and, unless my whole body says yes, I try to say no.

There are obviously some commitments in life that we must keep, but, wherever you can, try practising this. For this week, if it's not a full body yes, it's a no. The more you practise this and tune into your body wisdom, the louder and clearer you'll be able to hear it guiding you in all decisions you need to make.

INVOKE THE GODDESS

Hecate governs boundaries and is the Goddess to call upon when you need to set your own. She is also the Goddess of the crossroads and so will lend you her wisdom when you need to make tough decisions, life changes and decide which way to go next, which often requires strong boundaries.

She is considered one of the oldest embodiments of the triple Goddess reflecting her powers over heaven, earth and the underworld, and is often seen holding two flaming torches and keys.

Just as her origins are shrouded in mystery, Hecate has been associated with many different roles over the ages, such as the Goddess of the moon and the night, psychic work, witchcraft, protection, magic and divination. But she is perhaps best known for her part to play in the myth of the springtime Goddess Persephone, who was abducted and taken to the underworld by Hades. Hecate assisted Persephone's mother Demeter in finding her and guided them through the night with torches to bring her back.

Hecate leads us out of dark places, so call upon her when you are struggling with lack of boundaries, people-pleasing and falling back into old habits and patterns. Visualise her torches guiding you towards a life of more strength, courage and light – let her be your boundary beacon.

As a fierce protector and guardian, Hecate will lend you her strength and support to set and uphold your boundaries. As the Goddess of the liminal, the in between, she will help you to sit in the discomfort of your 'no's as you learn to create boundaries to make space for your 'yes's.

It's especially powerful to work with Hecate at night and during the dark phase of the moon, but she will show up for you any time you need her. If you're ready to have a boundary badass on your team, it's time to work with Hecate.

Create a Hecate altar

○   Create a sacred space where you can go to con-nect with Hecate and seek her guidance. You may include two pillar candles to represent her torches, perhaps a key as a symbol to being willing to unlock parts of yourself, and anything else that represents Hecate or boundaries for you – perhaps even a pic-ture of yourself to remind you that boundaries are an act of self-love.

○   Write down the boundaries that you are working with and keep them on your altar. Light your candles each day and read your boundaries to Hecate asking for her strength and support in setting and maintaining them, while keeping your heart open. Each time you set and uphold a boundary, celebrate this at your altar space and thank Hecate.

Leave lunar offerings

As a Goddess of the moon, offerings were left for Hecate during the dark phase of the moon. Continue this ancient tradition by leaving your own offerings for her in the days running up to a new moon. This is the lowest energetic and emotional point of the lunar cycle and, as the dark moon draws you deep into your emotions, it's usually this time of the month that you will feel the most emotion, frustration and anger, especially around those places in your life where boundaries are being overstepped/need to be set.

Over the nights of the dark moon, leave an offering for Hecate each night, such as food, flowers, something from nature or a crystal, and ask for her help and support in any life areas that you are struggling with.

On the new moon, get clear about what boundaries you want to set in your life over the following month.

During the waxing moon (as the moon gets bigger), ask Hecate to lend you her strength and courage to set and maintain your boundaries, and let yourself begin to show up and speak up.

As the moon wanes, Hecate will support you in having difficult conversations, strengthening your boundaries and letting go of your own boundary fears or anyone or anything in your life that is no longer serving you, which will become more obvious the stronger your boundaries get.

Burn away your boundary fears

○ Find a pillar candle that represents Hecate's torch (you can use one from your altar). Write down all the things you fear most when setting a boundary, then read these things out to Hecate and ask for her strength, wisdom and courage. Set these things (safely) alight visualising Hecate's torch burning them all away.

You can do this each time you are being challenged to set a new boundary and new fears arise.

○ You may also close your eyes and visualise dropping your fears and doubts into Hecate's torches, and even visualise her fire within you burning away the inner voices and fears that arise around your boundaries.

Alchemise your 'no' into a 'yes'

As the queen of witches and magic, Hecate can help you to alchemise your no into a yes. Each time you stand strong and say no to something, visualise Hecate taking that no into her magical cauldron, see it go up in flames and transform into the space for a yes and something new to come in for you.

As well as keeping things out, Hecate also holds the power to allow access and let things in, so let Hecate know what you would like to invite into your life to fill the space you are creating with your boundaries. She holds the keys to the gates of all realms and will help you to unlock parts of yourself as you stand firm in your boundaries, sense of self and what you truly want. Feel her celebrate with you each time you set a boundary and unlock a new part of yourself.

Embody the Archetypes

The mother

Call on your inner mother to hold and take care of you on your boundary journey. Just as a mother would fiercely protect and do what was best for their child, feel your inner mother protecting, nurturing and supporting you.

The wild woman

Call on your inner wild woman when you need to step out of what is expected of you and begin to walk your own path. Boundaries are often necessary when we begin to change, and that triggers those who want us to stay the same.

Draw Your Boundaries

When you need to set boundaries, you can try visualising them like a physical force around you. You may see yourself surrounded by a glass dome, white light or see the boundary written in the air between you and the other person.

You could also call on Hecate and visualise her using her torch to draw a boundary line between you and other people or see her standing in front of you creating a doorway that she doesn't let certain things or people pass through, like your own personal boundary bodyguard.

AFFIRMATIONS TO RECLAIM YOUR BOUNDARIES

○ 'I honour myself by honouring my boundaries.'

○ 'It is safe for me to create and maintain boundaries.'

○ 'I have the right to make decisions that are best for me.'

○ 'Saying no to others allows me to say yes to myself.'

○ 'I trust the wisdom of my body.'

I truly hope that this chapter has helped you to begin to honour yourself and your needs, listen to the deep wisdom within and begin to show up and stand in your power and truth. Let's take this new-found strength and use it to begin to heal the witch wound and the sister wound.

'Know that you no longer need to hide to survive. We need you and your gifts, power and magic.'

Chapter 4

RECLAIM THE WITCH WITHIN

As we continue our journey along the Goddess Path, I want to explore some of the deeper, ancient, subconscious wounding that gets in the way of us being able to fully embody, express and know ourselves, other women and the Goddess. Get ready to dive a bit deeper now as we look at the feminine wounds.

The Witch Wound

One of the main things that gets in the way of women truly embodying and walking the Goddess Path is something known as the 'witch wound'. The witch wound is an inherited, collective trauma that is buried deep in our psyche and our DNA. It is carried from our past lives and through ancestral lineages, from times when women were persecuted, shamed and even killed for being healers, wise women, wild women, herbalists, visionaries and truth holders.

Not so long ago, women like you and I would have been burned at the stake or drowned for the beliefs we hold around spirituality. During the witch trials, thousands and thousands of women were killed for what we are doing right now – connecting with our feminine wisdom, communing with nature, working with crystals or herbs or astrology, gathering to worship the moon, trusting our intuition or simply standing out from the crowd. This is what makes us fear being different or 'too much'; it's what prevents us from doing what we are being called to do; it stops us speaking and shining and sharing our gifts, and keeps us small and hidden and afraid.

I truly believe that one of the reasons many of our sisters were accused or burned was because they were untameable, uncontrollable, connected to their deep intuition, magic and knowing, and walking the Goddess Path. It was to silence them and their feminine gifts and powers, which were a threat to the powers that be.

Many of the accused women were older or single, which is why I believe that we fear getting older and often feel terrified at the prospect of not having met someone or got married by a certain age. This goes deeper than current societal expectations – it touches the ancient deep fears within us that we are vulnerable, unsafe and open to accusation. On the other hand, many of us remain almost eternally single, as it wasn't safe to be around us in ancient times, as you too may have been accused. We try to protect others from getting too close by subconsciously pushing them away. We carry this deep belief that there is something wrong with us and getting too close to us is harmful.

Women were killed for being too beautiful, too ugly, too outspoken, too confident, for turning down the advances of men or for daring to be different to what society said – sound familiar? Even today, much of the same witch-hunting goes on.

I know that I was burned at the stake in a past life; it is a knowing that I carry deeply in my bones. In the beginning of my spiritual journey, I'd hide a lot of what I was doing as there was a deep-rooted fear that it somehow wasn't safe for me to tell people about it. Around the same time that I started working with the Goddess, I became fascinated with the Pendle witch trials (as it happened close to my hometown in Lancashire). I remember visiting Pendle and reading the stories and feeling as though I knew the place and the women. The more I started to share about my spiritual journey, the more fear would arise within me about speaking out about such things as moon magic, intuition and crystals. There would be a voice within screaming at me not to talk about them and, as such, over the years, I know I've played small because of this voice.

I remember once being in the back of a taxi and trying to record Instagram stories about a heal the witch wound workshop I was running. I literally could not get the words out of my mouth in front of the taxi driver. Each time I'd get to the same part of the story, it's like my throat would close, my body would seize up and I felt a visceral fear about saying the words out loud. Even writing these words, there is a part of me that wants to delete this whole page and never speak of it again, as it doesn't feel safe. A survival instinct kicks in, I want to run and hide, shrink myself, silence myself, censor myself – but no more, I reclaim the witch within.

If you've ever found yourself feeling the same when speaking about your spiritual journey or the Goddess Path, if you know you have more to offer but you feel afraid and doubt yourself or your gifts, if you fear speaking the truth, or struggle to listen to and trust your intuition, or you just feel the truth of these words in your blood and bones, I invite you to also reclaim the witch within.

Reclamation ritual

The first part of this is to acknowledge the existence of the witch wound and how it plays out in your life. Take some time to journal on where you shrink, silence and censor yourself, and why. Is there a part of you that feels it's unsafe and that you need to shrink back into the crowd and hide yourself and your innate feminine wisdom and gifts? Do you have trouble trusting your intuition or feel afraid of your psychic gifts and when you just 'know' something? Do you hide your spiritual practices and beliefs or crystals from others for fear of being ridiculed or judged?

Look at how these wounds have benefited you and 'kept you safe'. Realise that these witch wounds have been working so hard to not only keep you safe, but also keep you alive. Now thank these wounds and let them know that you don't need them anymore, that you are going to reclaim the fullness of your magic, power, gifts and worth.

Next, do that. If you were going to fully reclaim your witch, what would that look like for you? Would you speak up more about your spiritual journey, embrace your witchy practices and beliefs, no longer be afraid to be single, not hold back your truth, begin to share your gifts, or trust and follow your intuition?

Know that you no longer need to hide to survive. We need you and your gifts, power and magic. Reclaim all that was taken from you and do it now for those sisters who lost their lives and can no longer do it for themselves. In their memory, commit to reclaiming the witch within.

INVOKE THE GODDESS

Hecate is the Goddess of witches and magic who we met in the last chapter. She is known to give her blessings to witches, passing on her wisdom and knowledge, and showing you the truth of how powerful you really are. Call upon her for your witch work and ask for her guidance, protection and wisdom to help you to fearlessly connect to and reclaim your witch.

She has strong ties to herbalism, psychic work, manifestation and working with the moon and nature, so call on her if you want to reclaim and develop any of these gifts. Visualise her using her keys to unlock your inner witch and free your magic and power. Ask her to become your teacher and offer yourself to her as a dedicated student – to be clear here, you do need to be dedicated.

Hecate will push you beyond your boundaries and into reclaiming the fullness of your witch. The original meaning of the word witch in old languages was 'wise' or 'wisdom', so reclaim the word witch and reclaim your wisdom. Know yourself as a witch – a wise woman connected to her wisdom and wild feminine power. Explore how the word feels in your body and as you speak it out loud. Begin to once again embody and feel the witch within as you reclaim your medicine woman, wise woman and wild woman with Hecate guiding the way.

Ragana is a Baltic Goddess of witchcraft, whose name literally means witch or to see. It is said that she often hides away or shapeshifts, is most active at night and does not like to be seen by strangers, and so she is the one to call upon if you are hiding yourself, your gifts or your spiritual practices.

You must be serious about your witch work for Ragana to reveal herself to you, so begin, as she does, in quiet devotional practices to your witch work. Get committed to your craft, your beliefs and your inner witch, as it's through this inner connection that you will find the confidence to begin to share more of it with the outside world.

As she begins to reveal herself to you, ask Ragana to help you reveal more of your true self to the world. Ask her to teach you and show you what she knows and listen to the tasks she gives you and the wisdom she imparts.

Isis is the Egyptian Goddess of magic, healing and protection. Pray to her and ask her to heal your witch wounds and look after you as you begin to share more of your magic with the world. Isis very often shows up in dreams, so pay attention to your dream world when working with Isis.

As a Goddess of past lives, sit in meditation with Isis and ask her to help you see and heal the witch wounding of your past lives so that you may now share your gifts freely. Ask her to show you the lessons that these lives offered and to help you to set yourself free from the past-life memories and fears that are now holding you back. Feel her healing, love and support alongside you as you reclaim your magic.

Embody the Archetypes

The medicine woman

Call on your inner medicine woman to show you any ancestral healing that needs clearing around the witch wound. Ask her to then show the many lives you have lived before in service when you were aware of your powers and magic, and to help you to reclaim and share your gifts once more.

The wild woman

Ask your inner wild woman to help free you of any past-life shackles of being suppressed, punished and denied for being who you were. Don't wait for permission to be all of who you are anymore – set yourself and your witch free, and embrace and celebrate your untamed wildness.

The Sister Wound

The witch wound has sadly led to the sister wound, which also lives in many of us. It is a deep-rooted pain or distrust we have towards other women. It shows up in comparison, insecurity and judgement, and often prevents us from feeling like we have a true sisterhood or that we can truly trust other women.

Centuries ago, women would gather for ritual and healing, to share wisdom and support each other. You've likely heard the phrase 'it takes a village', and, for our sisters of the past, that was the way that life was as women would also regularly cook, eat and raise children together in solidarity and support of each other.

We all know the incredible power of women coming together, and this was a threat to the patriarchal systems of control, especially during the times of the witch trials in the mid- to late-1600s. Groups of gathering women were accused of being in covens and these women were branded witches and killed. So women stopped gathering. What is worse is that an accused woman would often be encouraged to turn on and accuse another woman to save her own life.

The fear of gathering often lives on within us because of the danger associated with it, and pitting women against each other certainly lives on. Even now, we are constantly compared to each other and made to believe that other women are somehow a threat to us through advertising, body comparison, sensationalist cheating stories in the media where women tend to be blamed and TV shows where multiple women vie for the attention of one man. Rather than seeing other women as sisters and allies, we have been taught to see each other as competition.

We've likely all been disappointed, betrayed and hurt in relationships with other women as we continue to unknowingly play out these silent internalised patriarchal beliefs that women can't be trusted, we must somehow compete with each other and her winning means you losing. We may feel envy at another woman's success or relationship, or find ourselves constantly comparing our looks or body to another woman's. We may not feel enough in groups of women or that other women are somehow better than us or have everything that we want.

And as these feelings of insecurity, jealousy and judgement come up, we find ourselves pushing other women away thinking they may take something from us or shaming, gossiping about, excluding or putting them down. We only have to look at magazines or online gossip sites to see this play out in the larger world as attacks are launched (often by other women) on another woman's body, her relationship choices and career decisions. And when this happens, what do we call it? A witch-hunt. These wounds run deep.

Each time we tear down and censor another woman, we tear down and censor the Goddess herself. Each time we compete with or betray another woman, we betray and suppress the Goddess and ourselves. So, how do we put a stop to this?

It stops when we stop playing a part in it. When we realise that other women are a reflection of the Goddess just like us, and we come together once more instead of fuelling systems of repression and suppression and control. Because the truth is that women need other women; we need sisters, allies and community. We need to be able to see, feel, encounter and recognise the Goddess in each other, through each other. As we support and raise each other, we support and raise the Goddess and ourselves. Each time a woman wins, we all win.

If you truly want to walk the Goddess Path, it's time to reclaim sisterhood. And, as we do, we get to help each other, hold each other, heal each other and walk each other home along the Goddess Path.

Reclamation ritual

The first stage of reclaiming the sisterhood is to acknowledge that the sister wound exists. Journal on where the sister wound has shown up for you in your life – when you have maybe judged or criticised or shamed another woman or felt the same happen to you. Write down when you have felt less than or insecure around another woman and how that made you feel and act towards her.

Look at your own shadows (we'll do more of this in Chapter 7) and insecurities and how you project and judge, and work to heal these so that other women don't trigger you anymore.

In claiming where each of us has played a part in this ongoing wounding, we get to bring it to the light, say 'no more' and put a stop to it here. We stop fighting each other and instead start raising and supporting each other.

As part of your healing, you could write a letter to another woman (that you never need to send) to acknowledge where the sister wound played out for you in the past. You may choose to reach out and make amends in real life or by just calling that woman into your heart and mind and telling her all that you want to tell her. There may be cords that you wish to cut to release this energy (see page 119).

Next, start to reclaim the sisterhood. Commit to raising other women and seeing and accepting the Goddess in them. Commit to no longer gossiping or putting other women down. Gather in circles with other women, hear their stories, see the truth of who they are and, in turn, let your truth begin to shine through. Perhaps gather with friends and talk about your sister wounds, be vulnerable, share – this is how we heal this and come back together once more.

As women gather, especially with a shared intention, magic happens. We begin to remember who we truly are and the power of the divine feminine. We forge deep, meaningful connections and support and encourage each other through our vulnerabilities, fears, hopes, dreams and celebrations. This is sisterhood.

Ancestral Healing

I feel it's important to briefly mention ancestral healing here as so much of our feminine wounding is carried down through our ancestral lines in ongoing threads of conditioning, fears, unfinished business and beliefs.

You may have witnessed your own mother or grandmother suppress their voices, gifts or power due to societal or generational expectations, or witnessed yourself playing out some of their old beliefs and limitations, such as believing that only men can be successful and make money or if you do get a good corporate job, you should never leave to pursue a dream. You may have also found yourself to be the odd one out in the family, not quite fitting in and always feeling different – and that's because you have come to earth this time around to be the one in your lineage who does it differently. You are a cycle breaker.

Reclamation ritual

If you can, get to know your mum and grandmother's stories, their struggles and fears, and also what they hoped and dreamed and wished for themselves. You can connect further back in your lineage through meditation by visualising your ancestors sitting with you. Ask for them to make themselves known to you and share their stories with you. Add photos of your female ancestors to your altar and pray to them.

Each time you heal or grow or push beyond a fear or reclaim a part of yourself, tell your ancestors that you have done it for them, and you are healing your family line for future generations to come. You might visualise your family tree and send healing, light, forgiveness and love through all the branches, healing and clearing any pain and wounding in your lineage.

You are now nourishing the roots of your entire family tree. Each time you show up as all of you, speak up for yourself, claim what you are worth, overcome a limiting belief or behaviour, heal yourself or are the one to do things differently in your family, you do it for your ancestors past, present and future.

Isis helps us to remember our ancestral lineage and stories, so call on her to help you do this. When we begin to undertake our own healing, we get to heal our ancestral lineage and release inherited traumas and woundings that have been carried down. You get to do this work now for all the women who came before you who couldn't and no longer have a voice.

Healing Your Relationship with Yourself

Both the witch and sister wound work to prevent us from shining too brightly, embracing all of who we are and embodying the fullness of our Goddess energy, so let's close this chapter by looking at the relationship you have with yourself, as it's the most important one you'll ever have. The relationship that you have with yourself sets the tone for every other relationship in your life. How you speak to yourself is an indication of how you'll allow others to speak to you. How much you love yourself is an indication of how much you'll allow others to love you. As we explored in Chapter 2, your levels of self-worth and self-value will determine how you allow others to treat you.

If you want deep, true, authentic friendships and relationships, that begins by you showing up as all of you. Otherwise, people get to know the version of you that you think they want you to be, and those relationships can never have depth or real meaning. If you want others to really know you, you need to really know you. It's only when you begin to see and treat yourself as the Goddess that you are, that others will begin to see and treat you as the Goddess that you are.

I hope that through this journey you are already getting to know and love yourself so much more. I know it sounds clichéd, but you really do need to become your own best friend, lover, supporter and cheerleader, and give yourself what you are searching for in others.

Learning how to be in a relationship with yourself is one of the most powerful and life-changing things you will ever do, and it will deepen your relationship with the Goddess. Your soul came here to be uniquely you, to express what only you can express and offer to the world what only you can offer. Every dream, desire, want and need within you is there because it's part of what is needed in the world and only you can bring it to life.

Yet society, the patriarchy and these deep feminine woundings have tried to teach us that we are somehow not good enough just as we are. We have been judged, shamed, scrutinised and criticised for decades: too much, not enough; too sexy, not sexy enough; too quiet, too loud; too big, too small. We're told to wax and shave and pluck and try to live up to unrealistic and, quite honestly, unreal beauty standards to somehow feel we fit. When all that is really needed is knowing, accepting, embracing and loving every part of us for who we are.

All you ever need to be is YOU. All any of us and the world really needs is you showing up as all of you. We don't need a watered-down, censored, shrunken version of you. We need the Goddess you. And this starts by you showing up for yourself.

Show up for yourself

Showing up for yourself is such an important step in reclaiming your relationship with yourself as this simple act tells you that you can trust yourself and that you know that you are a Goddess worthy of your love, time, care and attention.

How often do you promise yourself that you'll start meditating or exercising or make a start on following a dream tomorrow, and then you find an excuse: 'I'm too tired, hungry, busy, [insert your excuse]. I'll start again tomorrow'? This is a form of self-abandon and self-sabotage, and every time you do this you tell yourself that you aren't worthy, you don't matter and that you can't be trusted.

Imagine if a friend told you they'd meet you for coffee tomorrow at 11am. When 11am comes round, they tell you they are sorry, they can't come, as they are too tired. But they'll definitely be there the next day. The next day comes around and once again there is an excuse – this time it's that they are too busy, but they promise they'll be there the next day. Then it's another day, another excuse. How long would you let this go on for before you stopped believing in and trusting them?

Each time you do this to yourself by not showing up for yourself you make it hard to trust yourself, and this impacts on your levels of self-worth and your relationship with yourself. You need to become your own best friend and be there for yourself, champion yourself, support yourself and really show up for yourself each day, making yourself and your wants, needs and desires more of a priority.

This is how you will heal the witch and the sister wounds as you get to know, love and trust yourself on a deep level, and no longer need as much external validation and approval and therefore no longer need to hide, shrink or compete.

Reclamation ritual

Commit to one thing this week that deepens your relationship with yourself. That may be simply placing your hands over your heart each morning and asking yourself how you feel and what you need. It may be committing to a daily half-an-hour of self-care that you do no matter what or who else tries to get your attention. It may be setting clear boundaries around someone's behaviour, as you know you are worthy of better/ different or having a daily journaling or meditation session dedicated to awakening the witch within or healing and strengthening sisterhood bonds.

As you commit to showing up for yourself each day, you'll begin to trust yourself enough to go after something brave and bold or take a step into the unknown as you'll know that, no matter what happens, you'll be there and you trust yourself to get through it. This will help you to know yourself and deepen your relationship with yourself and, in doing so, be able to face and heal any witch, sister or ancestral wounds that have been holding you back and keeping you small.

AFFIRMATIONS TO RECLAIM THE WITCH WITHIN

- ⭘ 'I reclaim my gifts, power, and magic.'
- ⭘ 'It is safe to be all of me.'
- ⭘ 'I no longer need to hide to survive.'
- ⭘ 'I am a witch.'
- ⭘ 'Sisterhood is safe.'
- ⭘ 'I see the Goddess in all other women.'

Through this chapter you have started to recognise, unravel and heal some of the deep wounding that keeps many women from knowing the fullness of the Goddess within us and all the women in our life. Let's now look at how you can start to reclaim the Goddess in your everyday life.

'Once you begin to devote your life to the Goddess and invite her into all that you do, your life will change completely.'

Chapter 5

RECLAIM GODDESS RITUALS

Our journey now brings us into quite possibly one of the most important parts of the Goddess Path. This is where you now begin to put into practice much of what you have learned along the path so far, and this is where you will begin to know the Goddess as your own.

One of the best ways to know the Goddess is through rituals and devotion. This brings a sacred element and meaning to your Goddess practice and will help you to connect to your inner world and strengthen your relationship with your inner Goddess.

Daily Goddess Rituals

So often in life we are waiting for this huge moment of transformation when we think everything will suddenly change, or the moment we find our elusive purpose somewhere out there, or we seek a grand awakening, quick fix or magical intervention from the Goddess. In truth, the biggest changes in our lives come from the little things we do consistently, daily. If you want lasting change and transformation in your life, what you do daily matters.

You can't say that you want to trust and believe in yourself and then spend all day berating yourself and telling yourself all that you do wrong. You can't say you want a deeper connection with yourself and the Goddess and then spend all day numbing out and avoiding. You can't say you want to know what your purpose is and then spend all day doing things that have no purpose and bring you no joy. You can't say you want something and to be someone and then do nothing to get it.

This is where you need daily rituals, which help you to dedicate and devote to what you want and who you want to be, and this is how it becomes your reality. It's in these daily touchpoints, where you connect to the Goddess and your soul, listen to your inner wisdom and take care of yourself, that bigger long-lasting change becomes possible.

In Chapter 1, we talked about creating a Goddess altar, prayers, journaling and affirmations, which I hope that you have been doing and have seen the benefits from. Let's now look at more daily rituals that you can create for yourself that will help you to connect more deeply to the Goddess to be able to hear her messages and embody her wisdom and energy. Be realistic about how much time you have to devote to the Goddess daily and then make sure that you commit to this time as a non-negotiable. The more you show up for her, the more she will show up in your life.

Listen to the Goddess within

The Goddess is feeling, emotion, understanding, and as you begin to listen to your inner world, the more you will hear and know the Goddess within. We'll look more at the power of emotions and intuition in Chapter 8, but, for now, begin by placing your hands over your heart each morning and asking yourself how you are, and then allow whatever needs to be there to be there.

Some days there may be sadness and others joy, overwhelm, grief, gratitude, answers or sometimes nothing at all. Hold yourself and your inner Goddess through whatever is present and allow it to flow through you.

Then ask yourself what you need today and let the answers come to you. Some days you may need to rest or be quiet or allow yourself to move gently with no big expectations. Others you may be nudged to speak your truth about something or set a boundary or show up and do something brave.

As you make a promise to the Goddess within of how you'll take care of yourself today, call upon the greater Goddess or any Goddess you may be working with for any help, support and guidance you may need, and feel her energy show up in your heart.

Invite her light into your life

Get a candle and dedicate it to the Goddess. Visualise this candle containing the divine feminine life force energy of the universe. Each morning, hold your (unlit) candle to your heart and feel the energy of the Goddess. Then, when you are ready, consciously light the candle as a way to invite the light of the Goddess into your day.

As you light your candle, say out loud, 'I invite the light of the Goddess into my day to light up the way.' Spend a moment or so gazing at the flame, the light of the feminine, and feel her energy and power.

You may also wish to whisper wishes, hopes and dreams, and anything you need support and guidance with into the flame.

As you blow out your candle, visualise giving all of these things to the Goddess so that she may support you and light and guide the way.

Devote your day to the Goddess

At the beginning of each day, devote yourself to the Goddess. You could do this after listening to the Goddess within or the candle-lighting detailed above. Ask her to weave her magic and guidance through your life and to awaken the Goddess within you. Ask her to show you how you can be of service and show up in the world as the Goddess that you are.

Then devote yourself to her all day. Devote all your actions, words, emotions and thoughts to the Goddess. Make everything you do through the day in service and devotion to her, even any challenges. See the Goddess in everything and make your life an offering to the divine feminine. The more you do this, the more you will awaken and embody the Goddess energy in yourself, and in those around you. Once you begin to devote your life to the Goddess and invite her into all that you do, your life will change completely.

Try a moving meditation

Whereas the masculine is stillness, stability and discipline, the feminine is creation, feeling and flow. This is why sometimes traditional seated, still meditations (although worthwhile) don't work as well to connect with the Goddess, who in her very essence wants to be free to move, weave and create. This is where moving meditations can be so powerful and help you to really begin to feel and embody the Goddess energy within.

1. Begin by standing with your feet slightly wider than hip-distance apart, soften your knees, let your arms hang down by your sides and gently close your eyes. Take a moment or so to just observe the movement of energy within your body and how you're feeling.

2. Begin to deepen your breath and breathe into your body, becoming aware of your inner world. Now, begin to feel for the Goddess energy within you. You may be working with Shakti, the divine feminine life force energy that we met in Chapter 1, and moving that through you today, awakening your own Shakti and inner Goddess, or you may be working with a specific Goddess or feminine archetype whose energy you can call upon.

3. Feel for her energy in your body. It may be a little bit of warmth or movement somewhere within or a feeling of love or power or pulsation. Focus on that feeling and allow it to get a little bigger and louder.

4. When you can really sense the Goddess energy within you, start to allow her to move you. She may want you to gently sway to begin with, with the movements becoming bigger and wilder the more you listen to her and follow her guidance. This takes some practice to begin with as you will keep finding yourself in your head questioning whether this is right or ok, or you trying to be the one who is doing the moving. Each time this happens, come back to centre, take a deep breath and find her energy again before letting her move you once more.

As you learn to allow the Goddess to weave, guide and move you in this way, this is the same way she will begin to guide you through your life, leading you towards where your soul wants you to go. The little inner nudge that guides you to sway, stomp, dance, shake and flow around your living room is the same guiding energy that will begin to let you know which direction to move in life.

When you can surrender to the guidance of the Goddess and allow her to flow and weave her magic through you in this way, your life will never be the same again.

Worship yourself

As you worship yourself, you worship the Goddess and begin to know and embody the divine feminine energy within you. This may be praising yourself often for things you do well or each time you do something brave and overcome a limiting belief or fear. It could be looking yourself in the mirror at the end of each day and telling yourself three things you did well that day.

One of my favourite ways to worship yourself and the Goddess is to get yourself some really beautiful body cream and, once a day, massage it into every part of your body, loving yourself fully. As you do, feel the touch of your skin, the feel of your body. Tell your body how beautiful she is. Get lost in the sensations and feel of your own body and worship yourself as the Goddess you are.

See yourself

Stand in front of the mirror, look at yourself and first notice if any judgements or struggles come up with this. Be kind and gentle and hold yourself through these moments. If you find yourself pulling parts of your appearance apart, pause, place your hands over your heart, breathe and connect to your inner Goddess, and then start again when you feel ready. See the image of the Goddess being reflected back to you and simply repeat, 'I see you, I see you, I see you.'

Then begin to gaze softly into your own eyes and allow your vision to soften and fade. Start to see 'beyond' the human you. As you gaze into your eyes, connect to what's within you – the essence of your soul, Shakti, the Goddess. Allow your soul to begin to rise within you and really spend some time connecting to the essence of you that is far greater than your physical body. Feel the love and acceptance that pours through you as you start to allow you to see yourself through the eyes of your soul.

Once you get comfortable with this, you can begin to do your moving mediation in front of the mirror. Dance for yourself, watching yourself. Let your Goddess move through you and watch how strong, sensual, sexual, powerful and wild she is. Notice how it feels and looks, and how you want to be touched. This may even end in a self-pleasure practice or just a practice about awakening and witnessing the Goddess within you.

Thank the Goddess

At the end of each day, say a prayer to your inner Goddess thanking her for her guidance and wisdom and always being there for you. Show your gratitude for all the ways she has shown up for you today and helped you. Ask her to show you anything that she needs you to see or know at the end of this day.

Ask for any answers or guidance or help you need, and ask for any issues you have had through the day to be resolved overnight, allowing your soul to work with you in your dreams. Feel a very deep connection with the Goddess and a deep trust that everything is happening exactly as it should.

Spend a full day in ritual

I'd also love for you to think about making a full day a ritual practice in motion: see your morning coffee as a ritual, eat your food as a ritual, see being in a meeting as a ritual, as though there is some divinely guided purpose that you are in that meeting at that time. See conversations with people as a ritual and using your voice as a ritual. See getting dressed as a ritual, movement as a ritual, a shower as a ritual, a walk as a ritual. Make your whole day and all that you do a ritual practice of connecting to the Goddess within you.

Deepening Your Goddess Rituals

Let's now look at some other rituals you can do to help you to let go of anything holding you back from fully embracing and becoming the Goddess that you are. As you begin to reclaim the Goddess once more, you will begin to make your whole life a ritual and offering and come up with many more rituals of your own.

Grieving ritual

As you take this journey along the Goddess Path, you may find grief arising when you realise how much of your feminine wisdom and power you have given away by never having been shown and taught this information.

We also don't grieve enough in life. We tend to save it for death, but in truth we need to allow ourselves to grieve all losses in life – such as the ending of things like relationships, jobs and friendships, dreams that you never followed and directions you didn't go in – as otherwise it's very difficult to let go and move on from them.

It can be hard to look at these things, especially those things we feel we missed out on. But if we don't allow ourselves to see the truth and grieve these things, they remain buried within us, affecting how we show up in the present and in the future. We get stuck in our stories and don't learn from these experiences and use that to move forwards in life into more of the Goddess we came here to be.

This is where a 'descansos' can be so powerful. Taken from *Women Who Run with the Wolves*, the work of the incredible Clarissa Pinkola Estés, this is a ritual where you give yourself a chance to mourn and grieve all the deaths and losses you have experienced in your life so that you can learn from them, release them and leave them where they are meant to be – in the past.

Through this potent ritual, you are honouring all the places and parts of your life where you felt a loss or when a part of you died, such as opportunities you feel you missed, times you didn't honour and value your worth or love yourself, disappointments and rejection you've experienced, heartache and heartbreak, the roads you didn't take, the dreams you didn't follow, the life you thought you'd have . . . and anything and everything in between.

Reclamation ritual

Here it is the descansos process in Clarissa's own words:

'I would like to introduce you to the concept of descansos as I've developed it in my work. If you ever travelled in Old Mexico, New Mexico, Southern Colorado, Arizona or parts of the South, you have seen little white crosses by the roadway. These are descansos, resting places. Descansos are symbols that mark a death. Right there, right on that spot, someone's journey in life halted unexpectedly.

'Women have died a thousand deaths before they are twenty years old. They've gone in this direction or that and have been cut off. They have hopes and dreams that have been cut off also. Anyone who says otherwise is still asleep. All that is grist for the mill of descansos.

'While all these things deepen individuation, differentiation, growing up and growing out, blossoming, becoming awake and aware and conscious, they are also profound tragedies and have to be grieved as such.

'To make descansos means taking a look at your life and marking where the small deaths, las muertes chiquitas, and the big deaths, las muertes grandotas, have taken place.

'I like to make a timeline of a woman's life on a big, long sheet of white butcher paper, and to mark with a cross the places along the graph, starting with her infancy all the way to the present, where parts and pieces of herself and her life have died.

'We mark where there were roads not taken, paths that were cut off, ambushes, betrayals and deaths. I put a little cross along the timeline at the places that should have been mourned, or still need to be mourned. And then I write in the background "forgotten" for those things that the woman senses, but which have not yet surfaced. I also write "forgiven" over those things the woman has for the most part released.

'Descansos is a conscious practice that takes pity on and gives honour to the orphaned dead of your psyche, laying them to rest at last.

'Be gentle with yourself and make the descansos, the resting place for the aspects of yourself that were on their way to somewhere, but never arrived. Descansos mark the death sites, the dark times, but they are also love notes to your suffering. They are transformative. There's a lot to be said for pinning things to the Earth so they don't follow us around. There is lot to be said for laying them to rest.'

I hope that after completing this powerful practice you can bury some things and leave them behind in the past, and learn from these past experiences to do things differently going forwards.

INVOKE THE GODDESS

Ceridwen is the Goddess to call upon for help with grieving and letting go. Through experiencing deep pain, loss and grief herself, she is able to hold and comfort us through our own. Part of her story shows us that, on the other side of grief and healing, there is hope and new beginnings.

She is the keeper of the cauldron of knowledge, transformation and change, and so visualise placing all of your grief and pain into her cauldron so that you may find the lessons and healing and transmute this into a rebirth.

Forgiveness ritual

In a similar way to grief, holding on to resentments, anger and pain from the past only causes more pain and keeps you trapped in an endless cycle of repeating the same stories and patterns. This is where forgiveness rituals can be so powerful, for both you and others.

Remember that forgiving does not mean saying that what someone did to you is right or ok. It means saying that you are no longer willing to carry it around with you and allow it to affect you and your life and keep you from experiencing the fullness of the Goddess.

Reclamation rituals

Forgiving yourself

One thing that keeps us stuck in a lack of self-worth and disconnected from our Goddess energy is constantly punishing ourselves for things we did wrong or didn't get quite right in the past. This can often keep us in a shame spiral, which causes us to doubt our worth, believe that we don't deserve good things/anything better and cause us to self-criticise and self-sabotage and not be able to move forwards in life.

Forgiving yourself means understanding that you can't change the past, learning from your mistakes and knowing that you did the best you could with what you knew at the time.

Begin with acknowledging and accepting what you did and why. Get really honest. Understanding your motives helps you to understand yourself on a much deeper level and understand why what happened happened. Then focus on what you learned from the situation, how you could have done things differently and how you will do things differently moving forwards, knowing what you now know.

Hold yourself, wrap your arms around yourself and say it: 'I forgive you.' Look yourself in the eyes in the mirror and say it out loud: 'I forgive you.'

Know that if you learned from it and commit to making changes and doing things differently in the future, you don't need to keep beating yourself up for it. You deserve your forgiveness; so free yourself to move on.

Forgiving others

Write a list of all the people who have done something to you in your life and then, one at a time, call them up in your mind's eye and say to them 'I forgive you.' Feel the forgiveness in your heart and then see them dissolve/walk away as you release them from your life.

INVOKE THE GODDESS

Rhiannon is the Goddess to invoke if you need help with forgiveness. A Celtic Goddess of healing, transformation and rebirth, Rhiannon too was once wronged and now teaches us the healing power of forgiveness.

Rhiannon shows us how to remain strong and courageous in difficult times and that the way to sovereignty and freedom is forgiveness, and that it's through this that you can begin again on your own terms.

Gratitude ritual

Hold a gratitude ceremony for all that has gone before you and all that has happened in your life so far as it has all brought you here, to this moment, where you have the power to make change. Gratitude is some of the most powerful, life-changing medicine that you will ever take.

Write a list of all the people, experiences, lessons, highs, lows and everything that has happened in your life that you have to be grateful for. Go through each thing on the list one by one and thank them/it for what it taught you and how it's made you who you are.

Birthday ritual

Celebrate yourself on your special day by writing a letter to the you of last year. Write about all the lessons you have learned, the challenges you have faced, the growth you have experienced and what you are most grateful for. Then write a letter to the you of next year telling her all your hopes, wishes and dreams for her, all the ways you'll support her and everything you want to create and bring to life through her. You can even put the letter to one side for now and post it to yourself to arrive on your birthday the following year – or schedule an email letter to arrive on your special day.

Rite of passage rituals

You may also want to consider rituals for each turning point in a woman's life (these will be covered in Chapter 11) with a menarche ritual for when a girl has her first period, a blessing way ceremony for mothers-to-be and a croning ritual for menopause.

AFFIRMATIONS TO RECLAIM GODDESS RITUALS

- ○ 'What I do daily matters.'
- ○ 'I devote my days to the Goddess.'
- ○ 'I dedicate myself to what I want and who I want to be.'
- ○ 'I listen to my inner world.'
- ○ 'I allow the Goddess to flow and weave her magic through me.'
- ○ 'I make my whole life a ritual and offering.'

You are now beginning to invite the Goddess into your life, allowing her to walk alongside you and weave her magic through you. Make your life now an offering to the Goddess and you will see such huge changes. Let's look now at how to reclaim your energy so that you can feel the energy of the Goddess much more easily.

'As you reclaim and refine your energy, you are able to access your intuition, inner wisdom and knowing, and your inner Goddess so much more easily.'

Chapter 6

RECLAIM YOUR ENERGY

Our journey along the Goddess Path now takes us into the stage where I'm going to show you how to reclaim your energy. Everything is energy: you, your thoughts, words, emotions and everyone and everything around you.

When your energy gets blocked, it can leave you feeling stuck in life, giving away your power, repeating patterns, replaying the same emotions, worries, fears and behaviours over and over again, and feeling disconnected from yourself and life, lost, drifting and alone.

You may feel constantly burned out and exhausted, struggle to set boundaries, keep being pulled back into the past, suppress your feelings and authentic self-expression, lose your motivation and creativity and shrink, feeling like you have nothing to offer to the world.

When you keep your energy clear, balanced and protected, you come into more of a natural flow and can begin to access, feel and know your intuition, inner wisdom and knowing, your inner Goddess and all the Goddesses and feminine archetypes so much more easily.

Let's look at how you can begin to consciously work with your energy and call upon the Goddesses to help you to clear, heal, balance and align your energy.

The Chakras:
Awakening Your Energy Centres

The chakras are energy centres in your body through which Goddess or life force energy flows. Each one corresponds to a different physical, emotional, physiological and spiritual aspect of your wellbeing. The word translates to 'wheel' in Sanskrit and, as the name suggests, chakras are spinning vortexes of energy that are constantly receiving, processing and redistributing information and energy from your inner and outer world.

When your chakras are balanced and in harmony, Goddess energy will flow freely through your body. However, through things like lifestyle choices, past experiences, suppressing emotions, pushing against life and living in constant stress, your chakras can become blocked, stagnant or overactive, preventing the feminine life force energy from flowing freely through you. This is where you can call upon some Goddess power to help you to realign these energy centres and bring yourself back into a place of balance, self-knowing and presence.

Have a look through the list below and see if any of these energy centres stand out to you, or any of these Goddesses call to you. You can also close your eyes and visualise each chakra one by one, checking in for any signs of imbalance. This method takes patience and practice, but over time, as you connect to you and your energy more, you'll have an inner sense of where you are out of alignment and what's needed to bring yourself back.

Root or Muladhara chakra

Located: at the base of the spine
Colour: red
Element: earth
Energy: I am

Your root chakra is responsible for you feeling safe, secure and at home in yourself and the world around you. It governs your basic needs for survival and connects you with the earth and an ability to stand strong and confident in who you are.

When it is out of balance, you may experience low self-esteem or self-sabotaging behaviours. You may become needy or insecure, and often feel anxious, unsafe or abandoned. You could also experience being flighty and ungrounded or, at the other extreme, stuck in your ways, afraid to make changes in your life.

INVOKE THE GODDESS

Call upon **Gaia** to balance your root chakra. Gaia is the Greek Goddess of the earth and the ancestral mother of all life. When you feel overwhelmed, anxious or disconnected from yourself, go outside into nature and lie on the earth. Invoke Gaia and feel the great mother holding, supporting and nurturing you. Or try standing barefoot on the grass and imagine sending roots deep down into the earth, feeling Gaia anchoring you into safety. Give Gaia any worries, stresses or concerns, and feel her take them into the earth to be transmuted. Then visualise drawing stability and security up from the earth into your body.

Goddess wisdom for your root chakra

Use the affirmation 'I am' daily. Stand with your feet rooted on the earth (outside if you can) and repeat 'I am safe and at home in myself.' Or if you are working on self-esteem and standing strong in your sense of self, say your name – 'I am Kirsty Gallagher' – and really allow yourself to feel and own the presence of who you are. Any time you feel yourself in overwhelm or anxiety, repeat 'I am safe, I am safe, I am safe' and feel the energy of Gaia holding and supporting you.

Goddess affirmation: 'I allow Mother Gaia's grounding, nourishment and safety to flow through me.'

Sacral or Svadhisthana chakra

Located: in the lower belly
Colour: orange
Element: water
Energy: I feel

Your sacral chakra is the home of your emotional, creative and sexual energy. It is responsible for helping you to be in feminine flow with life and able to express your wants and desires. It governs pleasure, desire, fertility and your ability to fully enjoy life.

When it is out of balance, you may struggle to connect to and trust your emotions and find yourself having frequent intense emotional reactions. Expressing your wants and needs will be difficult, as will trusting and flowing with life and connecting with your divine feminine. You may struggle with pleasure, intimacy and sex, either overindulging or avoiding them all together.

INVOKE THE GODDESS

Invoke **Oshun** to balance your sacral chakra. A Yoruba water Goddess of femininity, fertility and sensuality, she is associated with fresh, flowing water. Oshun teaches us how to flow and embrace sensuality, pleasure and prosperity. Call upon Oshun and imagine her sacred waters flowing through you, cleansing and clearing any blockages and awakening the creativity and sensuality within you.

Goddess wisdom for your sacral chakra

Check in at the beginning of each day with how you are feeling. Place one hand over your sacral chakra, take a few deep breaths and then say, 'I feel . . .' and say what you are feeling. Some days that may be 'I feel nothing' and others you may feel sad, anxious, happy, abundant or grateful. Begin the practice of tuning into your emotional world and what you are feeling. You could also add to this practice by allowing your emotions to move through your body. How would sad move? Would you gently sway your body side to side? Would anger stomp or joy jig up and down? Let yourself express what you are feeling (we explore more of this in Chapter 8).

Goddess affirmation: 'I allow Oshun's sensuality, pleasure and creativity to flow through me.'

Solar plexus or Manipura chakra

Located: in the solar plexus (between the rib cage
and belly button)
Colour: yellow or gold
Element: fire
Energy: I can

Your solar plexus is your place of personal power, individuality, courage and self-confidence, and the place from which you manifest your desires. It governs your sense of self, ability to shine in life and trust in yourself to go after what you want.

When it is out of balance, you will likely feel powerless and not in control of your own life, possibly always feeling like the victim and as though nothing good ever happens to you. You will struggle to assert yourself, believe in yourself and take action on your dreams. There will be a lack of self-confidence and a lot of self-doubt.

INVOKE THE GODDESS

Call upon **Durga** to balance your solar plexus chakra. We met this powerful Hindu Goddess in Chapter 1, and we now call on her again to help you to stand strong in your power, know who you are and let your inner light shine. Stand in power pose (feet hip-width apart, hands on hips, chest out, shoulders back and chin up) and feel Durga's strength and power coursing through you. You may visualise her letting out an almighty roar from within you that vibrates through your solar plexus.

Goddess wisdom for your solar plexus chakra

With Durga's help, do one thing a day that challenges you and helps you to take control of your own life and destiny. That may be working towards changing a habit or limiting belief, pushing yourself out of your comfort zone, setting a boundary, making a decision or standing up for yourself. Tell yourself often that you can do this, because believe me when I tell you that you can.

Goddess affirmation: 'I allow Durga's strength and power to flow through me.'

Heart or Anahata chakra

Located: in the heart
Colour: pink or green
Element: air
Energy: I love

Your heart chakra relates to all matters of love, both giving and receiving. It not only relates to love of others, but also self-love and your relationship with yourself. It governs compassion, trust, inner presence and peace, and relationships.

When it is out of balance, you will struggle to give and receive love, both to others and yourself. There is often a lack of self-love and self-care, and feelings of being unlovable and lonely will come often. There can be a big fear of rejection, causing you to further close off your heart. You will struggle to trust yourself and others or have weak emotional boundaries.

INVOKE THE GODDESS

Invoke **Aphrodite** to balance your heart chakra. As the Goddess of love, beauty and pleasure, Aphrodite will begin by teaching you to love yourself, as it's only from here that you can begin to love anyone else. First, open your heart to Aphrodite, allow her in and feel her energies infuse and begin to heal and open your heart. In times when you are struggling with love, rejection or taking care of yourself, place your hands over your heart and feel Aphrodite filling you with her love, strength and presence.

Goddess wisdom for your heart chakra

Create a daily self-care ritual for yourself that you devote to Aphrodite. This may be a skincare routine, meditation, evening bath, walk in nature or anything that says self-care to you. Mark this time out as sacred, as time spent in devotion to Aphrodite so that she can show you how to honour yourself as the Goddess that you are.

Goddess affirmation: 'I allow Aphrodite's love and healing to flow through me.'

Throat or Vishuddha chakra

Located: in the throat
Colour: sky blue
Element: sound or space
Energy: I speak

Your throat chakra is how you express your unique self out into the world. It gives voice to your heart, your wants, needs and desires, and your inner truth. It governs communication and expression. It is from your throat that you speak your truth into being and create your reality with your words, so begin to use them wisely.

When it is out of balance, you will struggle with communicating clearly and have trouble finding the right words or saying what you truly mean. You may be afraid to speak your truth or speak up, especially in public settings. On the other hand, you may find yourself gossiping often, telling white lies or speaking unkind words.

INVOKE THE GODDESS

Maat, the Egyptian Goddess of wisdom, truth and cosmic order, can be called upon to balance your throat chakra. Touch your throat and call on Maat when you are struggling to find the right words, speak up for yourself or express your needs, and feel her energy clear and open your throat so that you may speak your truth from within.

Goddess wisdom for your throat chakra

Find a beautiful essential oil blend (frankincense, peppermint or cypress are all good for the throat) and anoint your throat daily. As you place a drop of oil on your throat, call on Maat and say out loud, 'It is safe to speak my truth. I express my authentic self with ease', or any other words that resonate with you around healing and opening your throat. Commit to perhaps speaking only the truth for a week, or expressing what you need even when it feels scary.

Goddess affirmation: 'I allow Maat's truth and wisdom to flow through me.'

Third eye or Ajna chakra

Located: between and just above the eyebrows
Colour: indigo or purple
Element: light
Energy: I see

Your third eye chakra connects you to your intuition and wisdom, and is often referred to as the 'eye of the soul' as it helps you to see what cannot be seen with the physical eyes but is just known. It governs inspiration, visualisation and the ability to choose your own thoughts.

When it is out of balance, you will struggle to be able to hear or trust your intuition or anything that cannot logically be explained away. You may have a lack of self-knowing, unable to trust yourself and your own inner wisdom. You may also find yourself constantly overthinking everything or stuck in ego and being a bit of a know-it-all.

INVOKE THE GODDESS

Invoke **Hecate** to balance your third eye chakra. Hecate can see the past, present and future all at once and, as such, is all-seeing and all-knowing. When you are in times of doubting your intuition and inner knowing and unable to see the way forward, call on Hecate. Visualise her placing a finger on your third eye, opening your spiritual sight.

Goddess wisdom for the third eye chakra

Meditate on your third eye for a few moments every day. Call on the Goddess to help you to see what you need to see and know what you need to know. Pay attention to any flashes of insight or awareness that come during that time or during the rest of the day. Make a commitment to follow any intuitive nudges that you receive.

Goddess affirmation: 'I allow Hecate's all-seeing spiritual sight to flow through me.'

Crown or Sahasrara chakra

Located: at the crown of the head
Colour: violet or white
Element: spirit
Energy: I know

Your crown chakra connects you to the spiritual realms and helps you to receive wisdom and guidance from cosmic consciousness and the universe or divine. It governs higher awareness, life purpose, spirituality and connection to all of life.

When it is out of balance, you will very often struggle to find meaning in life or feel like you don't have a purpose or part to play. You may be sceptical, narrow-minded or feel very alone in life. You may feel like life is against you and frequently lose faith or hope.

INVOKE THE GODDESS

Call upon the divine Goddess herself, **Shakti**, the source of all Goddess energy, to balance your crown chakra. Feel her energy flow through you to help you to balance your crown chakra. As you connect to the divine feminine and awaken the Goddess energy within you, begin to access your true inner source of power and the life force energy of the universe that flows through everything.

Goddess wisdom for your crown chakra

Connect with the Goddess within you daily. We looked at ways to do this in Chapter 5. As you begin to awaken your own divine feminine energy and open yourself to accessing a whole new world of power, potential and purpose, you begin to know and live as the embodiment of the Goddess and all of who you came here to be.

Goddess affirmation: 'I allow the divine Goddess energy to flow through me.'

Balancing Masculine and Feminine Energies

We all have a blend of masculine and feminine energies in us. Masculine energy helps us to do, achieve and plan. It is protective, logical, helps us to get from A to B and gives us reasoning, willpower and focus. Feminine energy helps us to flow, receive and feel. It is intuitive, creative, helps us to trust in the flow and gives us receptivity, expression and manifestation.

Ideally, as women, we want to live in approximately 80 per cent of our feminine so that we are connected to our intuition, feelings and flow, with 20 per cent masculine, which we can tap into to help us to motivate, take action, set boundaries and stand up for ourselves when we need to.

When our masculine and feminine energies get out of balance and one becomes overly dominant, we begin to feel out of alignment, depleted, exhausted, stuck, lost or disconnected, to name just a few. In short, you'll just feel 'off' and the more you learn to feel and flow between these energies within you, the quicker you'll know which one is out of balance and needs some attention.

When you are too much in your feminine

When you are too much in your feminine, you tend to self-sacrifice, self-abandon and revert to people-pleasing and putting everyone else's needs above your own. You may struggle to make decisions, doubt yourself at every turn and have trouble moving forwards in life, being productive or getting things off the ground. You may get lost in your emotions, unable to rationalise them, or find yourself keeping it all in and then having emotional outbursts. There is a tendency to feel unsafe in life and become co-dependent and unable to do things for yourself.

How to invite in more masculine energy

Make a plan: This might be a simple daily to-do list or a plan for the week or month ahead. You might also want to spend some time looking at what you want for your life longer term and planning for that and how you will get there.

Set boundaries: Especially boundaries around your time and energy and carving out more time and space for you. See these boundaries as a way of you stepping into a protection role and taking care of yourself and your needs. (Revisit Chapter 3 for more on reclaiming your boundaries.)

Take action: Rather than just thinking about doing something (or overthinking all the different options and doing nothing), take action. Do just one thing, take one step, make one thing happen and this will start to build more confidence and motivation to keep going.

Create a routine: Although the feminine is all about flow, too much flow can leave us feeling unanchored and directionless. This is where a routine can give us that sense of structure, foundation and safety. This could be a simple morning or evening routine that keeps you grounded daily.

INVOKE THE GODDESS

Call upon **Athena** when you need more strength, power and courage. Athena is the Greek Goddess of war and wisdom. Known for her strategies, inventions and victories, she is a beacon of female empowerment. Call on Athena when you need discipline or focus, strength or protection, or when you need to fight for yourself or something you want. Visualise her standing alongside you ready to go into battle with you, lending you her courage or perhaps lending you her wisdom and helping you to plan and strategise your way forward.

When you are too much in your masculine

When you are too in your masculine energy, you tend to get stuck in the hustle, always switched on, doing, pushing and goal-chasing. You may shut down your emotions, unable to deal with them, and begin to question and doubt your intuition, needing proof or logical explanations for everything. You tend to be overly competitive, putting huge expectations on yourself and pushing yourself too hard, never allowing yourself any downtime or space to rest and switch off.

You will likely become controlling and hyper-independent, feeling as though you have to take care of it all by yourself, and struggling to ask for help and support. This is a common problem for single women/mothers or women business owners and entrepreneurs, as you do need to be the one taking care of everything and there is a weight of responsibility, but being too much in your masculine all the time is exhausting and leads to burnout and a sense of overwhelm and isolation.

Even though this comes from having to exert too much of your masculine energy, part of being able to surrender back into the feminine is by consciously asking the divine masculine to come in and take care of you for a short time so that you can surrender back into feminine softness for a while.

Let yourself be held by a bigger energy – call it God or universe or whatever name you choose – so that you don't have to do it all alone. Give anything you are struggling with up to a higher source of power and feel that you are being supported and held by something greater. Knowing that you are being taken care of, you then have the space to invite in more of your feminine energy.

How to invite in more feminine energy

Spend more time being: Whereas the masculine is the 'doing' energy, the feminine is the 'being', so make time to just be. This may be time in nature with no phone, a day with no agenda or strict plans, but doing what you feel like in each moment, or time to simply switch off, rest and receive.

Allow yourself to receive: This may be receiving the intuitive nudge that wants to come through when you get quiet and still enough to listen or receiving the gifts of your labour and enjoying the results of what you have been creating. Make sure, too, to receive help from others when you need it. Notice if this is something that's hard for you, as this is a sign of being stuck in your masculine, and commit even more to asking for what you need.

Spend time in nature: Nature is overflowing with the feminine life force energy, so head there when you need to reconnect. Get your bare feet on the earth, lie on the grass, swim in the sea or hug a tree. All these things will help you to reconnect to the feminine life force energies and the Goddess within.

Create, move and flow: The Goddess is not static or still; she is alive, weaving, moving, flowing. So, if you've been stuck at a desk or in your own head or in a state of doing for too long, move it out. Shake, dance, move, express and let the feminine life force move and flow through you. You can also try writing or painting, or anything that gets you out of your head and into your body.

INVOKE THE GODDESS

Saraswati is the Hindu Goddess of wisdom, knowledge, speech, learning, creativity and the free flow of consciousness. She can be invoked when you need more intuition, flow, expression and feminine wisdom. Her name means 'flow', 'fluid' or 'she who possesses water', and so call on Saraswati and feel her feminine creative waters flow through you. Feel her cleanse your mind of the hustle and struggle; feel her open your heart to receive and feel; allow her divine feminine energy to move and flow through you, awakening your creativity, intuition and your own inner wisdom. Let her Shakti show you how to awaken yours.

Releasing Energy Cords

Energy cords are invisible cords of energy that attach you to people, places and even things. They are formed through an emotional connection or reaction and continue to allow energy to flow between you and the other person.

While not necessarily a bad thing (think of the mother–child bond), cords can drain you of your energy and keep you stuck in the past, stopping you from moving forwards.

If you can't get over your ex, find yourself constantly thinking or speaking about someone in a negative or obsessive way, feel stuck and unable to make decisions about your future or find yourself wallowing in deep or unexplained emotions, it may be time to cut some cords.

Cutting cords helps us to let go of the past and take back our energy and power from anywhere that's draining it. It gives us autonomy over our energy and helps us to release anything that we no longer need from our lives.

It's not only the past that we need to cut cords with, but you may also sometimes need to cut cords in your current relationships to keep the energy clear and flowing. Cutting cords with someone doesn't mean cutting them out of your life altogether, but just that it clears the energy between you, almost like a reset.

INVOKE THE GODDESS

Call upon **Kali** to help you to cut energetic cords. The Hindu Goddess of time, life, death, creation and destruction, Kali helps you to release attachments, take back your power and transform your life.

Sit quietly, close your eyes and take a few long, slow, deep breaths. Invite in Kali's energy and ask for her help to remove cords that are holding you back and keeping you stuck and small. Kali is fierce, and so you may feel her presence quite strongly.

You may know who you want to cut cords with, or just be open to anything Kali wants to show you. If you know the person or situation, hold them in your mind's eye. Now, feel where in your body this cord is – it may be your heart or somewhere else like your left shoulder or hip; trust whatever comes to you. Thank whoever/whatever these cords came from for the lessons, but let them know you don't need them anymore and are no longer willing to carry this energy.

When cord cutting, I prefer not to visualise cutting, but rather untying. So, visualise untying or undoing the cord from your body and giving it to Kali. Feel her take it back to where it came from or destroy and transmute that energy, releasing it all together. Do this as many times as necessary and be sure at the end to thank Kali for her assistance. You may spend a little more time with her at the end allowing her to impart any wisdom and/or energy she wants to give you.

Clearing Your Energy

You can also work with your aura to clear your energy daily to keep your Goddess energy aligned and flowing, especially if you feel that you have been taking on other people's energy or leaking yours to them.

Your aura

Your aura is an energy field that always surrounds you and reflects your current emotions, thoughts, feelings, desires, sense of self and so much more. Our aura is our first point of contact with the world, and it is often auras that we pick up on when we are with others. You know how you just know someone is off without them having to say anything? Or how you may feel upbeat and filled with energy after time with some people and drained and exhausted after time with others?

Your aura is also an energy boundary that helps you to keep other people's energy out and protect your own. Just like the chakras, our auras can get clogged up with emotions, thoughts and limiting beliefs, and get depleted when we give too much of ourselves and our energy away, leaving us feeling drained and vulnerable. That's why it's so important to keep your aura and energy clear and strong.

INVOKE THE GODDESS

Isis, the great healer and Goddess of magic and protection, can be called upon to help you to awaken your own innate healing powers and keep your energy and aura cleansed and clear.

Begin by visualising your own aura. Ask Isis to help you to see and feel it. See if it is close to you or far away and whether there are any colours in your aura. Now, start to check for any stuck energy, emotions, thoughts or beliefs in your aura and ask Isis to help you to clear them away. She may dissolve them away with light, you may see yourself in an Isis magic rain shower cleansing it all away or you may feel her energy sweeping through your aura clearing away all that's no longer needed.

Next, begin to look for any holes or tears in your aura that may be leaking your energy or leaving you open and unprotected from the energy of others. These can often be formed when you self-abandon or try to numb out and 'leave your body' when things get too much. Ask Isis to help you to heal and seal these holes, filling them with her healing magic and light.

Finally, ask Isis to fill your entire aura with her healing energy. You may visualise light, colours and Isis's magic and power filling your aura. Decide how close you want your aura to be to you, and then ask Isis to help strengthen it and your energetic boundaries, feeling them strong around you.

Check in with your aura daily over the next week and keep calling on Isis whenever you need to heal and clear your aura or strengthen your energy boundaries.

AFFIRMATIONS TO RECLAIM YOUR ENERGY

○   'My energy is clear, balanced and protected.'
○   'I call my energy back to me now.'
○   'Feminine life force energy flows freely through me.'
○   'I bring myself back into balance and alignment.'
○   'My energy boundaries are strong.'

You've now learned how to clear your energy so that you can allow the divine feminine life force energy to flow freely through you, awakening more of the Goddess within. With our energy balanced and protected, let's now spend some time in the underworld, continuing our journey into your shadows and meeting the Dark Goddess.

PART 2
THE UNDERWORLD

We've now reached the midpoint and the doorway to the underworld. Before we enter, I want you to pause to check in with whether you are ready to take this next part of the journey – for once you've met the Dark Goddess, there is no going back.

There can sometimes be fear around meeting the Dark Goddess as you can't hide anything from her, and she will show you what isn't working in your life and where change and transformation need to happen. Often, we like to pretend that we aren't aware of these things as then we can avoid them and don't need to take the often difficult steps of making change. But that's what the Dark Goddess is here for.

She will demand that you step into your power, see your shadows and face your truths. She will help you to go where you've previously been afraid to go. She will push you to your limits, challenge you and change you – and you need to be ready.

So, take a moment here to think about your journey along the Goddess Path so far. Grab your journal and a pen, perhaps light a candle and some incense, and reflect on the following:

○ What have been your biggest realisations so far on this journey, about yourself, your life, the feminine?
○ How is your relationship with the Goddess? How is she showing up for you in your life? Where are you most feeling her support, guidance and wisdom?
○ How have you and your life changed since starting this journey?
○ What are you enjoying most about this journey and what are you finding the most difficult or challenging?
○ Are you ready to meet the Dark Goddess? What do you hope she will show/bring you? Are there any fears around meeting her?

Journal this out, then sit, place a hand over your
heart and one over your belly, and ask if you're
ready. Once you hear your full-body yes, it's time
for you to meet the Dark Goddess ...

'The Dark Goddess knows all that you are and all that you are capable of, and she wants to help you to claim it.'

MEET THE
DARK GODDESS

Frequently misunderstood, the dark feminine has often been seen as negative and something to be feared, but it is through working with the Dark Goddess that you will transform and heal your life.

We've been taught to fear the night and the dark, but at one time women ruled the night and the moon. Medicine women, wild women, witches – they were uncontrollable and connected to a much deeper source of power that didn't fit the cultural standards that were being created, and so, as we saw in Chapter 4, this side of femininity was suppressed.

Over time, women in their Dark Goddess energy were labelled witches, hags, sluts, disrupters and troublemakers, and women were only celebrated for being gentle, agreeable and passive. Femininity, as defined by patriarchal standards, was often seen as fragile, demure, submissive, sweet, obedient and very often weak – especially as women over the ages have been taught to silence and suppress themselves, behave in a ladylike manner and be the 'good girl'. In truth, it's only when you recognise and reclaim your dark feminine alongside your light feminine that you will truly liberate and free yourself.

When you embrace the light feminine, you reconnect to your intuition, feelings, emotions, grace, receptivity, compassion, ease, flow and nurturing. When you embrace the dark feminine, you reconnect to your power, passion, sexuality, authenticity, creativity, magnetism, courage, ferocity and magic.

If you're ready for this, if you're ready to enter your depths to know and reclaim all of yourself, if you're ready to walk alongside the Dark Goddess, let's descend . . .

The Wilderness

The descent into the underworld to meet the Dark Goddess usually begins with what I would call the void, or the wilderness. The void or the wilderness are times in life when we feel lost, directionless and lacking in purpose or enthusiasm for life. We feel like we no longer know who we are and what we want, and what we used to want no longer holds the same appeal. It can last for anything from a few days to a few weeks, and many people panic in these void times, as it can feel confusing and unsettling, especially if you are questioning everything in your life and nothing makes sense anymore.

But this journey into the void is very often the Dark Goddess calling, wanting to shake you out of your slumber and prevent you from sleepwalking in the wrong direction through your life. She wants to show you where you're dimming yourself, moulding yourself into someone you're not and denying your brilliance, for the Dark Goddess knows all that you are and all that you are capable of, and she wants to help you to claim it.

Wandering the wilderness is a time of such magic and potential – for it's in this space where there is nothing, that anything is possible. It's very often when you feel the most lost that you are actually finding yourself. In these times, you are no longer who you were, but you're not yet who you're becoming, and it's in the in between – the void – that the biggest amount of Dark Goddess magic can happen.

Anyone who knows me well knows that, a few times a year, the Dark Goddess calls me, and I visit the wilderness, the void. I do it now willingly rather than having to be dragged there. I feel it as a sense of discontent creeping in, sometimes deep loneliness; a sense of not knowing who I am, what I want or what I'm doing. I feel utterly lost. I find intense emotions coming from nowhere, and no ritual, mantra or positive thinking can shift me from it.

If I'm honest, when I look back, this usually comes at a time when I have been disconnected from myself, hiding, dimming myself, not following my intuitive nudges or gripping on to things that are no longer working for me, rather than trusting the process and allowing them to fall away.

After many years of fighting this, I now surrender to it. Rather than allowing the Dark Goddess to stalk me for weeks, I go all-in and turn to face her. When those familiar feelings start, I take the fast-track lift to descend down into the underworld. I see this as a powerful opportunity to reconnect back to myself and to meet the Dark Goddess in all her glory.

First, I give myself a time limit. We never want to stay in the underworld for too long; we want to visit to gain what we need from there and then bring that wisdom back with us. It's usually a maximum of three days for me.

Second, I realise that I don't need a reason for how I'm feeling or to give it a story – it just is. I allow myself to be in the not knowing. I don't try to search for answers or reasons or stories or to solve or fix anything. I don't try to numb it away or eat it away or Netflix it away. I just surrender and allow it all, and know that this, too, shall pass and, when it does, a new me will emerge from the ashes of my past.

Third, I realise that this is a death and rebirth process; that a part of me and my life is dying away. I hold myself and allow the old parts to die away, creating space for the new to emerge.

Finally, I dance with the Dark Goddess. I invite her in. I ask her to be with me and help me to remove anything no longer in resonance and to show me the way. I get curious about what I am feeling, what's here, what's present. I give myself permission to feel everything I need to feel, and cry, laugh, rage, stomp, scream, breathe, move and process my emotions without labelling or making anything good or bad.

I allow myself to go to the depths of the darkness. I turn towards the mystery, the alchemy and the Dark Goddess. And I can honestly say that these are some of the most transformational times of my life, and I emerge as someone completely different on the other side.

Reclaiming Your Rock Bottom

Every heroine's journey has a rock bottom – a moment when they feel they just can't do it anymore. And this is the turning point of true reclamation.

You've likely experienced those moments in your life when you are on your hands and knees on the floor and simply don't know what to do. Or when it's felt like you can't take much more, or that your heart is going to break into a million pieces.

Yet it didn't. You're still here. You've overcome every hard thing in your life so far. And I'll bet that, when you look back on those times, you'll realise that they are the times when you learned the most about yourself and the moments that made you. Because it's in our rock bottoms that we meet the Dark Goddess.

Just as Shakti, the divine feminine, is creation, she is also destruction. The Dark Goddess is an agent of change, a bringer of chaos, a force to be reckoned with. In nature, she is the storms, tsunamis and volcanos, and it can often feel like she brings this same energy into our lives, especially when we are straying from our soul's path.

The Dark Goddess knows that it's only really when we are in the depths of despair or when our back is against the wall that we learn the most about ourselves and how strong and capable we are. It's in our darkest moments when we really get to know ourselves and are called to rise and be there to support, encourage, trust, care for and love ourselves.

I know that these hard times can feel unsettling and leave you feeling unsure of yourself, your faith and life. But these rock bottoms truly are some of the most powerful and transformational times of our lives.

While we can't always consciously choose what happens to us in life, we can always, always choose how we respond and react to what is happening. When you see yourself as a victim and that things are happening to you, you lose all your power and do become a victim of that circumstance. When you see life as happening 'for' you, everything changes. You begin to see the opportunities, growth and lessons in what you are going through and become an active participant in your own life, even if it feels challenging. You get to call upon the Dark Goddess for strength, help, support and understanding, deepening your relationship with her and yourself.

Anytime you notice yourself in a difficult situation or spiralling in your mind, ask yourself, 'What can I learn from this?' or 'What is this showing me?' Rather than allowing yourself to fall into victim, try to see the bigger picture, the teachings and the lessons, the way in which this is the Goddess showing you that you have moved out of alignment with your soul.

Sometimes, admittedly, the lessons don't become clear until a little further down the path, when you can look back and connect the dots. But by reclaiming your rock bottoms, the whole process of what you are going through will become a spiritual experience of honouring your soul's path and meeting the Goddess rather than of struggle.

When things feel like they are crumbling down and falling apart, I now know that things are actually coming together. It may be that I was travelling down a wrong path and my soul needed to redirect me, or that I'd been ignoring the niggles and nudges for too long and the Dark Goddess needed to get my attention.

I know that in these times I am being remoulded and, although that process can feel painful and desperate, these are the times when I learn the most about my own deeply held fears, insecurities and old programmes. These are times of transformation in which I am coming face-to-face with old identities, beliefs, thoughts, patterns and ways of being that are no longer serving me. I am being asked to crumble, surrender and let go of old constructs so that a new Goddess version of me can emerge.

But this comes with experience – when you can look back and see that every rock bottom has been a defining moment in your life that has helped you to get closer to where you're meant to be. So, let's do that now.

Reclamation ritual

Look back over the most difficult and challenging times of your life with the eyes of your soul. Journal on what these situations taught you, how you overcame them, how you grew, how they helped you to evolve as a human and a soul, and how they have made you who you are and brought you to this moment. See how far you have come and, most of all, that you have overcome every difficult situation in your life so far. Realise how powerful and capable you are.

If you could tell the version of you going through that hard time something, knowing what you now know, what would that be? Then remember this advice for future times and know that you will get through this, your soul chose it, the Dark Goddess is beside you and these are the moments that are making you.

Dancing With the Dark Goddess

The Dark Goddess is chaos and creation, death and destruction, uncontrollable and unknown, mysterious and magical, wild and untamed. She brings you face-to-face with what you need to see, hear and know, demands you speak your truth and asks you to uncover all that you have been hiding and repressing. She supports you to be brave, bold, fierce and true to yourself, shaking off the expectations and opinions of others. She is painful realisations, uncomfortable truths, radical authenticity and the place where transformation happens. She helps you to burn it all to the ground and then helps you to rise from the ashes as the most healed, powerful, magnificent version of you there ever was.

The Dark Goddess will often call to you in a way that you cannot ignore. You may find yourself thinking about her con-stantly, hearing her name as though whispered on the wind, meeting her in your dreams, feeling her energy close by or begin-ning to see her symbols everywhere. She can sometimes be hard to initially connect with, as she lives in the shadows, and she will only fully reveal herself to you when she is certain that you are ready for the journey that she will take you on.

Working with the Dark Goddess takes time, effort and energy. You need to build a relationship with her slowly, as it's only through the depth of this relationship that you will learn to know her, trust her and allow her to take you to the levels of transformation that she wants to take you to.

Begin by finding out more about her, study her myths and legends, know her story, her struggles, her power, her lessons and her archetypal energy. Look at where her story mirrors your own and how she could help you in your own life.

Next, introduce yourself to her. Let her know that you are ready to work with her. The Dark Goddess loves offerings, so you may light a candle for her each day or create an altar that represents her, or just spend a few moments each day in dedicated devotion to getting to know her.

Meditate on the Dark Goddess, invite her in and open yourself to receiving her energy and guidance. Journal to the Dark Goddess, telling her what you need her help with and be sure to also journal on any messages you receive from her. Begin to feel her energy weave itself through your life and start to follow where she wants to guide you.

There are many names that the Dark Goddess goes by, each with her own unique energy. Let's meet a few of these with some ways to invite in and consciously work with their energies. Each one may call to you in a different way, at a different time, but one thing is for sure – when the Dark Goddess calls, you listen.

Kali

As Kali, she is the destroyer, the fiercest form of the divine feminine energy Shakti. Kali is a Hindu Goddess with glowing dark skin and wild flowing hair who wears a necklace of skulls, a tiger-skin skirt and is usually seen with her tongue out. She is known for her legendary battle with the demon Raktabija, where she helped Durga by drinking his blood, helping to slay him and his army of demons.

Kali is the ultimate expression of Mother Nature. The Goddess of death and rebirth, she brings destruction so that there can be new creation. Kali will liberate and free you from your fears and all that holds you back. She tears down old belief structures, frees you from resistance, pushes you out of your comfort zone and helps you to face your inner demons.

Invoke Kali when you need to stand up and speak up for yourself, find the courage to face your fears or when you know you are stuck in limiting beliefs and hiding and holding yourself back.

Offer your doubts, fears and limiting beliefs to Kali. Imagine bowing before her and giving all that you no longer need to her. See her take it from you and destroy it, creating the space for something new to come in.

When you want to truly call in Kali's power, stick out your tongue and take an almighty roar, harnessing your inner Kali and the power within. You may even want to move, dance or stomp as you do this. Feel her energy course through you, freeing and liberating you.

Lilith

As Lilith, she represents rebellion, freedom, independence and equality. A Jewish Goddess, legend says that she was the first wife of Adam, created from the same soil and clay as him. A sexually liberated and empowered woman, she was unwilling to be subservient, submissive or considered inferior to Adam; she wanted to be treated as an equal. She asked Adam for this and, when he demanded that she live under his authority, she transformed into a screeching owl and left the Garden of Eden.

Lilith embodies sensuality, sexuality, freedom, untamed wildness, liberation and feminine empowerment. She is considered by many to be the first feminist as she fought for equality and independence. She is a trailblazer and a rebel, helping you to forge your own path, to not be afraid of your shadows or sexuality and to rise in your power.

Invoke Lilith when you have lost yourself, especially in relationships, or when you don't feel fully able to be and express all of yourself around others. She's also the one to call on when you need to put yourself first more or if you want to work with your sexuality and sensuality.

Practise mirror work, where you gaze at yourself in a mirror to see the true you. See beyond any stories your mind may want to tell you and see yourself in your full feminine power. When you get comfortable with this, progress to looking at yourself in a full-length mirror, building up to moving and dancing in front of the mirror, allowing yourself to be seen in your full, unbridled sensual flow as you move.

Look at where black moon Lilith is in your birth chart. In astrology, this represents your dark side and your shadows, where you have felt shamed, repressed, misunderstood or ridiculed in your life, and how that made you shrink and hide your feminine powers. She'll show you what you may feel afraid to express, your powers of seduction, how you defy conventions and how you grow from struggles to empowerment. Use this knowledge to set more of your inner Lilith free.

Hecate

As Hecate, she is the queen of the witches, medicine woman, Goddess of magic, crossroads, the night and the moon. A Greek Goddess, she was the only child of Perses, the God of destruction, and Asteria, the Goddess of falling stars and nocturnal oracles. Hecate was granted power over the earth, sea and sky, and the cosmic world soul. As a liminal Goddess and guardian of entrances, she also became associated with the underworld, especially as she helped free Persephone (see page 62).

Hecate represents natural cycles, your menstrual cycle, the moon, nature and major life transitions. She teaches us about the mysteries of life, particularly women's mysteries, blood mysteries, womb wisdom, fertility and midwifery. She is a triple Goddess, reflecting her power over heaven, earth and the underworld, or birth, life and death. She is a Goddess of divination, connecting humans with the spirit world and the universal source of all creation.

Invoke Hecate when you are at a crossroads in your life, feel like you have been in the void for too long or when you need to set clear boundaries for yourself. She is also the Goddess to call upon when you want to work with women's healing, moon magic, fertility and blood mysteries, and witch work.

Call on Hecate in meditation when you feel lost or at a crossroads. Visualise her armed with blazing torches guiding you out of the darkness. You may light a candle daily to represent Hecate's guiding light, ask for her wisdom and guidance to help you find your way, and then blow out the candle trusting that your wishes have been heard. Look out for Hecate guiding you and follow her.

Connect to your magic and inner witch/medicine woman. Find a set of oracle cards and dedicate them to Hecate. Each morning, tune into her energy and ask her what you need to know about your day, then pull a card to guide you. Spend some quiet time journaling or meditating on the message of the card, opening yourself to receiving Hecate's messages and mysteries. Hecate is known to speak through dreams, so pay attention to your dreams too.

Ceridwen

As Ceridwen, she is the shapeshifting Goddess of change, rebirth and transformation, who holds the cauldron of knowledge, transfiguration and inspiration. A Celtic Goddess of Welsh descent, she is mother to Taliesin, the greatest of all Welsh poets, but only after a long story that contains magical potions, an unthinkable accident and a lot of transformation, death and rebirth.

As the keeper of the magical cauldron, a central theme of Celtic mystery tradition, she represents the womb of the Goddess, from which all life comes into the world. When faced with a huge challenge and obstacles, Ceridwen didn't give up, teaching us how to keep going through tough times, and that it's through these challenges we transform and end up where we're meant to be.

Invoke Ceridwen when you know it is time for a change or to let things go that are no longer serving you. When the discomfort of staying is beginning to outweigh the discomfort of change, you know it's time to invite her in.

Hold a burning ceremony to release what you are ready to change and transform. Write a list of all that you are ready to allow to die away. Read the list to Ceridwen and ask for her courage and guidance and help to let these things go. When you are ready to release, safely set the paper alight and drop it ideally into a cauldron (or fireproof dish) and watch Ceridwen's fires of transformation burn it away.

Ceridwen represents the changing of seasons in nature and your own life, showing you there are natural cycles through which you transform. As the Goddess of astrology, Ceridwen helps us to see these times represented in our birth charts. Look out for your Saturn return (around the ages of 29, 58 and 89), Pluto square (between the ages of 37 and 43), Jupiter return (around the ages of 24, 36, 48, 60, 72, 84 and 96), Neptune square (between the ages of 40 and 43) and Uranus opposition (in your early forties). Ask Ceridwen to help you to understand and embrace these radical turning points in your life.

'When you claim, own, accept and love every part of you, it doesn't matter whether anyone else does.'

Chapter 7

RECLAIM YOUR SHADOWS

We've met the Dark Goddess and entered the underworld and it's now time to dive into your depths.

Shadow Work

I want to say right now, as we begin this part of our journey together, that shadow work is hard. So, congratulate yourself on taking this brave first step towards self-awareness and transformation. Also, shadow work is tricky as it, well, hides in the shadows, so, this is a longer-term process of continually noticing your triggers, projections, emotions and judgements.

Be mindful, too, that shadow work should only be done with mindful, kind, compassionate awareness and as a tool to love and accept yourself more, rather than another reason to beat yourself up.

If you are struggling with low self-esteem, start by working with the Goddess to build a sense of self-worth and acceptance first before you dive too deep into shadows or call on the Dark Goddess. Perhaps go back and work through the first few chapters of this book again and come back to the shadows when you are ready to bring them to the light.

The idea of the shadow came from psychologist Carl Jung. Put simply, your shadow is all the parts of you that you try to hide, suppress and deny. It's the parts of you that you judge, see as weakness, are embarrassed about, don't like, don't want to face or think are bad. It's your shame and all things about you that you believe aren't acceptable or loveable, or the things you fear if other people knew about you would make them no longer like you. It's all the ways in which you don't feel safe to be yourself.

Anything about us that doesn't align with the image that we want to portray to the outside world gets pushed into the shadows. It's the emotions, desires and beliefs that you fear to express, the words you're too afraid to speak, the wild, chaotic, untamed, out-of-control Dark Goddess parts of you who you don't allow to surface for fear of what she may say or do.

The best way I ever heard the shadow described was having to carry a watermelon around with you all day, but you couldn't let anyone else see it. Can you imagine for a moment how not only virtually impossible but utterly exhausting that would be? That's how shadow work feels – when we walk around all day everyday trying not to let others see or know or discover certain parts of us. Trying to constantly hide parts of you is exhausting.

The shadows hold such power over us as they stay hidden, and we are terrified of anyone else finding out about them. But when you turn on a light in a dark room, the shadows don't seem so scary anymore. When you claim, own, accept and love every part of you, it doesn't matter whether anyone else does. You're no longer spending your time and energy trying to be someone you're not. When a shadow is brought to the light, it loses its power.

When we own love and accept all of ourselves, we have nothing left to hide anymore and we can begin to live freely.

Many of the beliefs and ideas that cause our shadows have been given to us by usually well-intentioned caregivers in child-hood or handed down to us by society, which tells us how we should behave, speak and be. As we are shamed, told off or teased for cer-tain behaviours, we start to hide these parts of ourselves and adjust our behaviours to suit what we think others want and expect of us. For example, if you were told off for talking too much or too loudly as a child, the likelihood is that you buried that part of yourself and will struggle now to speak up for yourself. You may even be ashamed if you catch yourself talking too much or raising your voice and work to bury that part of you even deeper.

Or perhaps an ex told you that you were too needy and it was too much, and so now you repress that part of you and become unable to ask for help, get support or show any kind of 'weakness', trying to prove that you can do it all alone and don't need anyone. You will shame the part of you who needs anyone or anything and become someone who is perpetually ok, even when you're not.

One of the main ways that our shadows show up is in what triggers or bothers us. A trigger is when we experience an uncom-fortable, often strong, emotional reaction to something, and we experience it often when it comes to our shadows. Let's look at how we can work with those triggers to recognise our shadows.

Meeting our shadows in ourselves

The shadow is that little voice that follows you around. It warns you to be careful not to say that or they won't like you. Don't behave like that or they'll judge you. Don't show that part of yourself or they'll think you're weird. Don't act like that or they won't want you.

Your shadow will have you believing that you are too much or not enough. It tells you that you're not worthy, not deserving, not loveable. It gives you a constant little reminder that there is something wrong with you and that you need to hide that part of you from the world.

We also see the shadow in ourselves when we notice our triggers and reactions to what someone says about us, especially if we feel they are seeing or uncovering a part of us that we try to hide and not allow the world to see.

Let's stay with our example above around being shamed for talking too much or too loudly when you were younger. Then one day someone in your workplace or your partner says, 'Wow, you just talked on the phone for a long time didn't you.' And this defensive rage comes up in you because you feel that they have seen that part of you who you try so desperately to hide; that ugly, unworthy, unlovable part of you who just talks and talks. So, you defend and fight back: 'No, I didn't, I don't know what you are talking about. I wasn't on the phone for too long' as you desperately try to hide that shadow part of you back away.

It's important to mention here that no one can ever make you feel anything unless you give them permission to. We are only usually upset by something someone says about us if deep down we believe it to be true, especially if it's a shadow part of us that we are ashamed of or that we are trying to suppress and deny.

So, if someone called you selfish and you didn't believe yourself to be selfish at all, it would bounce right off you and there would be little to no reaction. If there was a part of you that believed you were selfish, as you'd been told that by family or past partners, and you didn't like or were ashamed of that selfish part or judged being selfish as being something bad, you would immediately leap into defence mode – 'I'm not selfish, you're self-ish, how dare you call me selfish.' If, however, you'd already owned and loved your selfish parts as you used it to set better boundaries, practise self-care and put yourself first when needed, their words wouldn't have too much impact and you may even proudly agree, as you'd claimed your selfish. It's no longer in the shadows, and you no longer need to fear others 'finding out' about your selfish.

This is how shadow work is so powerful and transformative. The Dark Goddess helps you to know, own, accept and love every part of you, and by accepting your shadows, it sets you free.

Reclamation ritual

Start a shadow journal. Become aware of the recurrent shadow thoughts and feelings you have about yourself and note them in your journal. Each time the little voice that tells you there is something wrong with you pops up, be aware of it and what it is telling you. Spend some time with these shadows: can you see where they came from or why you are trying to hide this part of yourself or what you feel it would mean if others saw this side of you?

Pay attention to your triggers and emotions and spend some time with them. Rather than just dismissing them and wanting them to go away, gently ask things like, 'What am I feeling, why am I feeling like this, where do I feel this emotion in my body, what belief is attached to this emotion, what does feeling this emotion make me want to do?' Ask yourself why you just did what you did or reacted how you reacted. Hold yourself gently and be honest. This is how you will begin to uncover more of your shadows.

Meeting our shadows in others

Our shadows can also show up for us in what we find triggering, difficult or distasteful in others, or what we shame and blame others for.

To stay with our previous examples again, we'll be really bothered by anyone around us who talks too much or too loudly, as we see in them something we have suppressed in ourselves as we believe it to be unacceptable or unlovable. And in doing so, we are unable to speak our truth, so we find it uncomfortable to be around someone who can so openly share their voice.

We'll be triggered by someone being selfish and saying no to us to put their needs first as we've hidden our selfish to try to be more likeable and available and a good girl and because being selfish is 'bad'. And in doing so, we always put ourselves last, which deep down doesn't feel good either and so it's uncomfortable to be around someone who puts their needs first.

Anything that you see in others that triggers or bothers you or that you judge, dislike or want to run from and avoid is likely a shadow being reflected back at you.

One of the biggest ways the shadow shows up is in the sister wound that we met in Chapter 4. We've likely all had a moment when another woman walks into the room and she's confident and bold and carries herself as if she truly knows and loves who she is. Or she is comfortable in her body and exudes sensuality and femininity and isn't afraid to be all of who she is. And our first reaction is often 'Who does she think she is?' or we may find ourselves silently judging and criticising or avoiding her. This is because she directly triggers the parts of us that we have hidden, because society or lovers or others in life have told us to shrink and not be too much or too sexual or too wild or too confident or too flirty or to love ourselves too much. Or we don't feel worthy or good enough and so are unable to feel that amount of love and acceptance and confidence in ourselves. We've shamed, hidden and suppressed so many parts of our feminine powers, sensuality and our inner Goddess, and we can't bear to see her alive in another woman.

In truth, every time you see something in another woman that makes you want to judge, shame or criticise her, this is an invitation for you to reclaim a lost, hidden and repressed part of yourself, and for you to rise as more of your true, authentic Goddess self.

Reclamation ritual

○ Watch your emotional reactions, triggers and judgements to other people, especially other women. It is sometimes easier to see your shadows in other people, as what we are seeing is a reflection of a part of ourselves that we find unlikeable or unacceptable or that we have repressed.

○ Make a note of what you judge or criticise other people for or what upsets and bothers you most about others or their behaviour. Notice what words, traits, behaviours and emotions have the most emotional charge for you – for example, if you can't stand selfish people or when people are angry or loud.

○ Spend time reflecting on what it really is about their behaviour that bothers you. Keep going deeper and deeper into the why, gently asking yourself why their behaviour has upset you as much as it has. Explore whether you can see any of the same behaviour in you or whether they are exhibiting something you repress that you need to reclaim. This can be done through an inner dialogue (asking yourself the questions above kindly and lovingly) or through journaling too.

INVOKE THE GODDESS

We met the **Dark Goddess** and some of her embodiments on pages 129–141. Let's now look at how we can invoke her to specifically help us with shadow work and, most of all, healing, claiming and owning our shadows.

Very often we create shadows around the dark feminine as we are taught these things are sinful, bad, unacceptable or wrong. This causes us to reject our emotions, desires, sexuality, independence, passion, power, wildness and any other parts of us that society doesn't deem acceptable or 'ladylike'.

This is why shadow work is so important, especially as it feeds directly into the witch wound, the sister wound and many of the reasons you can't show up authentically as the true you and truly set your inner Goddess free. This is where the Dark Goddess can help.

The Dark Goddess isn't afraid of any part of you – there is nothing you could tell her that would make her love you less. She will help you to unapologetically own parts of you and accompany you to face your shadows and, in doing so, claim and free all the Goddess within.

For it's often the things we are most afraid of that hold us back the most, yet also hold our biggest gifts. No longer fearing speaking too much or too loudly means reclaiming your voice and truth. No longer fearing being selfish helps you to put yourself first. No longer fearing being too needy helps you to authentically express your needs and ask for what you want. No longer fearing your sensuality and sexuality means embracing the fullness of your pleasure. No longer fearing your anger and rage means being able to reclaim your sacred no and set boundaries.

Reclamation ritual

Call upon the Dark Goddess to help take you into your own underworld to see what you are hiding, repressing and denying. You could do this in meditation by visualising the Dark Goddess taking you down into your depths, into the deepest, darkest places to meet your sacred shadow. Let the Dark Goddess show you what you are hiding and where you've denied the dark feminine, and ask her to help you to reclaim these parts of you.

You may have hidden your desires, rage, passion, sexual liberation, pleasure, power, sensuality, wildness, magic, intuitive knowing or anything else that society has taught you is not part of being a 'good girl'. Ask the Dark Goddess for advice or guidance and feel her bringing your shadows to the light. You may even visualise meeting and talking to your shadow self and gaining insight and wisdom from them.

It's important to mention here too the shadow or wounded feminine. The shadow side of feminine energy usually comes from us not feeling fully safe in our feminine energy and so we create a set of defence mechanisms and survival strategies to try to help us to get our needs met. These include manipulation, criticism, jealousy, co-dependency, being the victim, attention-seeking, people-pleasing, vanity, comparison, self-gratification, withholding love and judgement. Get honest about whether any of these show up for you, even if you try to hide them. See if you can discover where they come from and what these shadows are trying to gain or protect you from. It's only through radical honest reclamation of your whole self and bringing all of your shadows to the light that you can heal and free yourself.

You could also journal on your shadows. You can safely burn this paper afterwards if it feels too scary to keep it, and visualise the flames burning away these things and beginning to free you from them. Even bringing them to the light and claiming these parts of you means that they no longer lurk in the shadows and have so much power over you.

Notice each time one of these shadows shows up for you, or you find yourself repressing or hiding parts of yourself, and call on the Dark Goddess to help you to bring them to the light and set yourself free.

You could work with any of the Dark Goddesses mentioned on pages 136–141, or here are a few more.

Persephone

Spending half of the year in the underworld, Persephone is the perfect guide to show you how to bring your shadows into the light. Persephone embraces her shadows without losing her light and teaches you how to not lose yourself by being someone that others want you to be.

Nyx

Goddess of the night and the darkness, Nyx will help you to face your fears, uncover your deepest truths and stay safe in the darkness, no longer fearing the shadows. She will show you that your greatest potential is often born out of your greatest fears.

The Morrigan

Often thought of as a triple Goddess, the mighty Morrigan will help you to face your deepest fears, uncover all the parts of you that you have buried in shame and shape-shift your darkness into light.

Ereshkigal

Queen of the underworld, she is one of the ultimate shadow Goddesses helping you to go into deep self-reflection and discovery of the depths of your inner world and all that you have hidden to see the truth of who you are.

AFFIRMATIONS TO RECLAIM YOUR SHADOWS

○ 'I bring my shadows to the light.'

○ 'I love, own and accept all parts of myself.'

○ 'My shadows no longer scare me.'

○ 'Seeing my shadows sets me free.'

○ 'My shadows help me to reclaim a lost, hidden, repressed part of myself.'

I truly hope that through meeting your shadows and the Dark Goddess you have started to claim, love, own and accept all parts of you. This is where true healing happens, and you begin to fully embrace the Goddess within. Let's now ascend and take all that you have learned about yourself in the underworld and use it to reclaim your emotions and intuition.

PART 3
THE ASCENT

Now that we've been in the depths of the underworld,
the only way is up! Taking all that you have learned
on your journey so far, you can now begin to rise
into who you came here to be. It's time to
remember and reclaim the Goddess within and for
you to start becoming your most empowered self!

'Within you is the answer to every question and the solution to every problem.'

Chapter 8

RECLAIM YOUR EMOTIONS AND INTUITION

Our journey along the Goddess Path now takes us into your emotions and intuition, both of which are divine feminine superpowers and ways the Goddess will communicate and weave her feminine wisdom through you. They are your inner navigational system and, when you can learn to access, trust and follow them, you get a roadmap for your life.

Embracing Your Emotions

Let's begin with your emotions, as it's only through your emotions that you get to access your deeper intuition and knowing. Our emotions are messengers, signposts; they hold such powerful insight and information for us and are something to be honoured and accepted rather than suppressed and denied.

In fact, it's in the denying and suppressing of emotions that most of our issues around truly knowing ourselves come from.

As we deny our emotions, we deny the Goddess her expression and flow, and we also deny ourselves.

We may speak of wanting to be able to trust our intuition or to tap into that deep inner wisdom and knowing, but the truth is that every time we avoid, deny or turn away from an emotion, we avoid, deny and turn away from the well of deep inner knowing within us – our internal navigational system.

As we learn to sit with our emotions, especially the uncomfortable ones, and be with them, listen to them, feel them, express them and move them through our being, we are able to access the deeper wisdom that often remains trapped and unheard beneath layers of old, suppressed emotion.

One of the main problems with feeling your emotions, especially in our modern-day spiritual and manifesting world, is that we have been taught it's 'good' to feel happy, grateful, abundant, joyous or excited, and its 'bad' to feel sad, angry, lonely, overwhelmed or lost. This has been further compounded by the masculine world around us that is frankly terrified of the power of women's emotions and teaches us to hold back our feelings, suppress, deny and push them back in and carry on as normal. We have learned to become afraid of the depth of our emotions.

Yet the truth is that it's in many of our deeper, darker emotions that the truth lies as these are the emotions that show us where we are out of alignment in our lives, going against our values, not honouring ourselves and our worth, and what needs our attention and requires change.

We looked at reclaiming our rock bottoms when we met the Dark Goddess in Part 2. In a similar way, it's the more painful emotions that come along to get your attention, and it's only when the deep grief or loneliness or rage hits that we can no longer ignore what we have been avoiding.

I know that, at times, it can be hard to have to face what you are feeling, as with that comes the admission that something is not right and a knowing that you need to make changes or leave or do something uncomfortable that you've not wanted to face. But these are the moments when you get to take back your power and access the full guidance of your inner Goddess.

The Goddess teaches us to tap into the power of our emotional world and to allow our emotions to flow through us. Just as the moon embraces her ebb and flow, and this is where much of her power comes from, the Goddess wants you to tap into the power of your emotional world, allowing your emotions to flow through you so that you can feel their wisdom, express them and let them go.

Many of our issues with emotion come through not being able to express them, especially things like anger. We've been taught as women that good girls shouldn't be angry and, as such, when we feel anger, we tend to panic, swallow it down and try to avoid it. But all that happens then is it festers within us and tends to come out in explosive rage.

Anger is actually a beautiful emotion as it shows you where a boundary has been crossed or something has happened that isn't ok with you. It's an adaptive response to something that you feel is a threat. If you can learn to feel and express your anger in the moment, it helps you to be assertive, speak your truth, express your needs, know your worth and use the wisdom and guidance behind the emotion.

Let's look at some ways to begin to know and embrace your emotions. You may want to start here by taking some time to gently explore whether you allow yourself to feel your feelings and whether there are any emotions you are afraid of and why, or where you feel you have suppressed emotions in the past and why.

Reclamation rituals

Listen to your emotions

A beautiful daily practice to get into the habit of doing is to place your hands over your heart, close your eyes and allow yourself to go inwards and feel. What usually happens here is that a little bubble of sadness or anger may come up and, because we can't bear to sit in the discomfort of that, we panic, open our eyes, pretend it didn't happen and move on with our day. Or we question why we're feeling like that and list all the many reasons why we shouldn't feel sad or angry and, in doing so, invalidate and abandon ourselves and our emotions.

As mentioned earlier, we often only want to feel the good stuff, but you can't selectively feel your emotions. You can't feel joy, happiness and gratitude without also feeling sadness, loneliness and grief. You have to feel the fullness of your emotions, and it's in the witnessing of all our emotions that emotional alchemy happens, and you can begin to seek the wisdom in what you are feeling. So, try to simply witness your emotions without attaching a story to them or judging or questioning what you are feeling.

Allow the emotions to come up and name them if you can. It's important to remember to say, 'I feel' rather than 'I am'. You are not your emotions; they are simply messengers passing through. For example, 'I feel sad' – now just be there in the sad for a moment, don't try to push it away. See if it has a message for you, or whether it just wanted to be witnessed and released.

You may notice that when the sad has moved on, a little bubble of happiness comes up, and then some grief, and then some joy; just keep witnessing and allowing your emotions to flow.

If you haven't allowed yourself to feel your feelings for a while, you may be feeling and releasing something that has been stuck in there for a long time, and so there may be a lot of previously unfelt emotions coming up to be felt and released. Initially just be with whatever is present without needing to know where it has come from or understand it. Take your time with this process and the feelings that want to arise. The more you learn to know and trust yourself, the more quickly and easily emotions will flow through you.

Once you are used to this practice of feeling, you might begin to gently talk to your emotions seeing what they have to share with you and what they want you to know. Give them a voice and listen to their wisdom. This is not only a beautiful practice of self-awareness and self-knowing, but also self-trust and self-care. As you hold yourself through difficult emotions, you begin to learn that you can trust yourself to be there for yourself and not abandon or leave when things get hard.

I often self-soothe in times of big emotions. I'll put my arms around myself or gently rub my heart and, when she's hurting, let me know that I am here, and I've got me. Other days, especially if my heart feels numb or lonely, I'll whisper, 'I'm here, I'm listening' and let myself know it's safe to feel.

Express your emotions

When we don't allow ourselves to feel and express our emotions, they get trapped, stuck and stored in our bodies – we've likely all heard the term 'emotional baggage' and perhaps all know how it feels to carry around pain, resentment and anger.

Letting these emotions move and be expressed through you helps you to process and integrate them – and then release them so that they no longer stay pent up. To do this, find yourself a safe space, allow yourself to feel the emotion and then let the emotion begin to move through you. If you feel sad, how would your sadness move? How would your anger, joy, sensuality or jealousy move? This may be through swaying, rocking or stomping, or if you have a lot of built-up emotion, punching pillows can feel so good. See if you can let go and allow the emotion to express itself fully through you.

I have found music really helps, as does calling on the Goddess, and I've been known to rage dance, stamp my hands and feet and sob in a heap on the floor (sometimes all within the same session!). For us women especially, we have been taught to silence ourselves for so long that we can often have trouble using our voices. Let yourself groan, sigh, moan, howl and cry, and express the guttural emotions that want to be released.

Try shaking too. This is such a powerful practice to help release tension, energy and emotion. It is a natural response in the animal world to shake off threat and discharge the energy of fear and fight, flight or freeze, and we can use it to do the same. Start by maybe shaking your hands, then your arms, then your feet and legs, and then allow your body to shake in any way it wants, visualising that you are shaking off all that you no longer need.

You may also try expressing your emotions through creation. Rather than bottling them up or letting them consume you, purposefully draw, dance, paint, write or sing them out. Allow these emotions to be expressed and use them to help you tap deeper into your creativity and the ways in which the Goddess wants to move and flow through you.

INVOKE THE GODDESS

Invoke **Artemis** to embody and embrace your emotions. As a Goddess of the moon, she teaches us that, just like the moon, our emotions and energy will naturally ebb and flow and we won't be the same every day, nor should we wish to be. She will remind you of the wisdom in your emotions and that they are not a weakness, but powerful messengers to be honoured and explored.

Call on her to help you to cultivate a deeper connection to your emotions and what they want to tell you. As a Goddess of nature and the wilds, she will especially help you to embrace and express your deeper wild emotions that you may try to hide, showing you that there is wisdom in your wild.

Aligning With Your Intuition

One of the things I am asked about most often is intuition and how to access it, and what the difference is between your intuition and your mind – so let's start there.

The voice of your mind is loud, insistent and very often confusing as it swaps and changes its mind, often arguing for both sides, flipping between one thing and the other, yes and no, this and that. It uses a lot of words and questions, and doubts everything, and can sometimes be critical and fear-based, leaving you feeling even more uncertain.

The voice of your intuition comes from somewhere deeper within. It is quiet, calm and clear, and usually just uses one word. It's a feeling, a knowing, a certainty. But it takes time to get used to listening to and trusting this wise, all-knowing, loving presence within as we've been taught that intuition is rubbish and, if it can't be debated and understood with the logical mind, it's not true or real.

Taking back the power of our intuition is one of the most life-changing moments along the Goddess Path, and it begins with realising that your intuition very often won't make any sense to your logical mind. So much so that, over the last few years, I have started to live by the belief that the less logical sense it makes, the more I know to follow it. This is what it means to begin to live in feminine flow.

For example, a few months ago, I was given the opportunity to move to a different part of the country, which meant leaving London, my home for ten years. The place I was offered was up for sale, so it was temporary with no guarantee of how long I'd be able to be there before it sold. But something within me just said yes. Even though it made no logical sense to leave my entire life for a non-permanent whim, I just couldn't shake off the deep intuitive yes. So, I said yes, and I handed my notice in on my London flat without even seeing where I was going to move to. It just felt right. And since being here I have felt happier and more whole than I have done in a long time. I am living in full trust and surrender on a beautiful life adventure with the Goddess, trusting that I'm right where I am meant to be and that the rest of this journey will unfold just as it's meant to.

For the feminine isn't logic, spreadsheets or mathematics. She's deep inner knowing, body wisdom, feeling and flow, and when we can begin to trust that and allow the Goddess to guide us through our intuition, the more magical life becomes.

This begins by following simple nudges like calling or messaging someone who has kept coming into your awareness, or trusting the niggle that tells you to say yes (or no) to an invite, or taking the detour or the spontaneous weekend trip, or saying out loud the idea that has kept coming to you.

The more you learn to trust in yourself and your intuition, the more the Goddess will speak to you and ask you to take bigger leaps of faith and use your intuition to guide bigger life decisions.

I see intuition as the way that the Goddess guides us towards becoming more of who we came here to be and following the path that our soul wants us to take so that we can experience, learn and evolve in all the ways that we are meant to. Speaking of which, one of the other reasons we tend to ignore our intuition is that it will often tell you the things that you don't want to hear. Your intuition is the quiet voice that says 'leave' when, deep down, you know a job or relationship has done its time, but you are afraid and trying to convince yourself to stay.

The Goddess knows what's best for you and will challenge you to push beyond doubts and fears to listen to and trust your intuition – this is part of how you grow and begin to weave your life with the Goddess. She wants you in your fullness, potential and power, and will be the little niggle deep within telling you that something's not right.

Let's now look at some ways to begin to reclaim and listen to your intuition and inner knowing.

Reclamation ritual

Begin by reflecting on your past experiences with intuition. Very often, we learn to trust our intuition in hindsight by looking back on the times we did and didn't follow it. Think of a time when you went against a little inner niggle that you were feeling: what was the outcome? Then think of a time when you followed that little inner niggle, even if it made no sense: what was the outcome of that?

As we've touched on a few times through this book, the feminine wisdom of intuition and knowing lives in your body, not your mind. When you get that feeling of truly knowing something, it's usually deep down in your belly or womb space. We even say, 'I felt it in my gut' when we are talking about something that we knew deep down to be true. So, begin to listen once more to the wisdom of your body. Any time you notice yourself trying to think your way to a solution or going over and over something in your mind, try instead dropping your awareness out of your mind and into your body.

Get quiet, still and listen to the wisdom within. Get beneath the noise of your mind into your well of inner knowing. I truly believe that within you is the answer to every question and the solution to every problem, but we are just usually looking for them in the wrong places. Look within and *feel* for the answers within you. Start to notice over time where and how your intuition makes itself known to you – is it a feeling deep in your womb, a full-body yes, a little inner nudge that won't go away or a sense of swirling sensations in your belly?

The next step in reclaiming your intuition is to begin to follow what you are being shown so that you can begin to have lived experience of living by your intuition. No matter how well you learn to listen to your intuition, it won't make any difference in your life if you don't act on what you are hearing. Start small with this to build up trust, maybe just picking up the phone to someone when you think of them or following a nudge to go somewhere. The more you follow and trust your intuition, the more she will speak to you, so if a little voice says stand up in the middle of the day, stand up. If it tells you to cross the road, do it. The moment a little nudge or niggle comes to you, act on it. Notice if you start to overthink it and question it (that's the ego mind), and instead just follow what you are feeling.

I also live by the rule of three: if I hear about a place three times I go there, a book three times I read it; any time something makes itself known to me three times, I listen, trust and follow that guidance. It's how I ended up living in my last London flat and the story behind it is quite magical. I'd yet again handed in my notice on a whim and was trusting that the Goddess would guide me to where I was meant to be next, but with just a few days to move out of my current place, it was getting a bit close to the edge. Over the space of two days, three people mentioned Notting Hill to me, so I did a flat search in Notting Hill and fell in love with the first one that came up. I enquired and got a notice back that it was gone, and so sadly decided it wasn't to be. A few moments later I got a call saying it was still available. I went straight over to see it, took it and moved my things in a few days later, and lived there happily for three years. Life is quite magical when you learn to listen, follow the signs and trust.

Speaking of signs, look out for them as a way that the Goddess will begin to speak to you through the world around you. This may be repeating number patterns, billboard signs that give you the answer to a question you were just asking, synchronicities or seeing things in your dreams. Be mindful to follow these signs too, and not to fall into the trap of always looking for a signier sign! In the same way we doubt our intuition, so often we will ask for guidance, get a sign and then ask for another one or a bigger one or a more obvious one. Start following the signs and they will connect you to even more layers of deeper intuition.

Finally, make sure to celebrate when you follow your intuition and something happens. This is how you will really learn to begin to trust. Keep an intuition journal – note in here the times when you received signs and messages and when you followed them, and the times when you didn't trust or follow your intuition. Your intuition is like a muscle, and you need to keep strengthening it.

Just a little note here: we often confuse excitement with fear, as they both feel the same in the body. When we are about to follow our intuition into something brave and unknown, we tell ourselves that we are afraid, and it mustn't be right and so we shouldn't do it. But there can never truly be change in your life without a certain amount of fear because, as humans, we're hardwired to resist change. Also, if there is no fear in following your intuition or making change is easy, there is no growth, no learning, no evolution, no trust and no having to push out of your comfort zone – which is what your intuition often wants you to do as it nudges you towards everything waiting for you on the other side of the doubts and fears of your human mind.

Following your intuition means not letting any doubts and fears hold you back and, over time, finding enough trust and faith in yourself, the Goddess, your soul and the universe to know that you can follow your intuition, even if it feels scary and unknown. You begin to trust in what you are hearing and believe in your own inner wisdom and intuition, finding faith that you do have all the answers within you.

INVOKE THE GODDESS

Call upon **Saraswati** to help you to connect to, hear and know your intuition and wisdom. Her name means 'flowing one' and she helps you to access the deep knowing that wants to flow from within and through you. She will remind you that all the answers you seek are already within you, and that the wisdom you are looking for is beyond words or rational logical thought – it's a feeling, a nudge, a flow.

She will help you to begin to weave and flow through your life following your own internal navigation system, easily recognising the difference between your intuition and the voice of your doubts and fears. She will connect you to the intuitive flow that lives within you.

P.S. Above I told you the story about how I was offered somewhere to live that took me out of London, but it was up for sale. Well, when I was two days away from the deadline of this book, the 'worst thing' happened, and I was told it had been sold.

Human me went into panic mode. Not only was I under huge pressure to finish this book, but I was now going to need to leave where I was living, which I loved, and find somewhere else to go. It was a lot, and I crumbled a bit under the pressure.

But I realised that this was a chance to practise what I preached, to walk my talk, to live by my beliefs and truth, and to trust and surrender fully to the universe and the Goddess. I went into nature and called on her to please help me, to guide me, to show me the way. I prayed, I allowed my emotions and I leaned deeper into trust. I knew that somehow everything would be ok.

I decided to get the book finished and then sort out my living situation. That same day, my best friend sent me a place, more as a reassurance not to worry as there were other things out there. Something niggled me all day so I thought that, even though I wasn't meant to be doing anything but the book, there would be no harm enquiring, which I did.

I got a reply to say that they had just had someone else take it, but they would let me know if anything changed. I surrendered deeper into trust (and emotion if I am going to be totally honest) and that night I got a message to say it was available again if I was interested.

I went to look at it and loved it – the landlords are amazing, and I truly feel that this is the next step in my journey here and this is where the Goddess now needs me to be. It's all unfolding just as it should, and I am trusting and flowing and allowing it all. This is how the universe and the Goddess will take care of us when we trust.

What gets more magical about this tale is that, after I had been told the lodge was sold, I went for an evening walk and a deer walked across my path. It struck me as a sign and so I looked up deer medicine when I got home – 'Deer Spirit appearing in your life acts as a teacher of how to be gentle, determined and sure even in difficult situations.' They are also strongly connected to the heart chakra, and this felt like a beautiful affirmation to be gentle with myself, trust and keep my heart open.

The following morning, as I was on my way to the woods, three deer walked across my path – I could hardly believe that I was witnessing these messengers again. Then, when I went to look at my new place, the landlady was telling me all about the beautiful woodland walks all around the house and she said to me, 'I even saw six deer on my walk the other day.' The deer had shown up for the third time and, in that moment, I knew I was taking the house and said yes without hesitation.

AFFIRMATIONS TO RECLAIM YOUR INTUITION

○ 'I trust my intuition and deepest knowing.'
○ 'I listen. I take guided action. I trust.'
○ 'I trust my intuition more each day.'
○ 'Everything I need is already within me.'
○ 'I am wise, intuitive and all-knowing.'
○ 'The Goddess speaks through my intuition.'
○ 'I follow my own internal navigational system.'

I hope that at this stage in our journey you are beginning to know and trust yourself so much more and allow the Goddess and your intuition to guide you towards even more magic and meaning in your life. Let's use this inner guidance to now begin to know and reclaim your truth.

'Speaking your truth means sharing yourself authentically and truthfully from your heart, with no second-guessing, censoring or fear.'

Chapter 9

RECLAIM YOUR TRUTH

We're at the stage of our journey together now when we're going to reclaim your truth. It's time to get raw and real, honest and vulnerable with yourself and see what you need to see, hear what you need to hear and know what you need to know. If you're ready, let's begin.

The Truth of What Needs to Change

After all that you have experienced so far, and meeting yourself in your shadows, it's time to face the truth about what is no longer working in your life and what needs to change.

We spoke about change in the last chapter, and how it's almost impossible without some kind of fear. I know that change feels scary, and it can often feel easier to stay in your comfort zone and avoid it, but that is not living, it's existing, and the Goddess wants you to live. So, what intuitive nudges have you been avoiding? What have you been resisting? Where do you need to face the truth? For only the truth will set you free.

One of the first ways to create change is to accept our part to play in things that aren't working in our lives, which I know can be difficult. But while we continue to make it someone else's fault that we are unhappy or can't have what we want or are unable to move forwards, we have to wait for that person or situation to change before we can change.

As soon as you accept radical responsibility for your part to play, you take back your power over the situation and reclaim the power to change it. For example, maybe you've been unhappy in your relationship as your partner doesn't value your worth and treat you in the way that you want to be treated. As such, you are always sad, don't feel good about yourself and spend a lot of time thinking, 'If they would just be nicer to me then I could be happy' or 'If only they'd change then this could be a good relationship.' You could likely sit and tell me a hundred things that they have done wrong and all the ways in which their behaviour affects your life and question all the reasons why they won't be nicer, more loving, more caring or just give you what you need.

But the only question that you really need to be asking is, 'Why do I stay?' Is it that, deep down, you don't believe that you deserve any better, or you are afraid to leave, or that you worry you might never meet anyone else? As soon as you accept responsibility for your part to play in allowing yourself to be treated in this way and accepting and settling for less, you can then take back your power to begin to make the necessary changes within you to know what you deserve and ask for what you want. The person in question will either be able to give that to you or they won't, and, at that point, you'll have found enough of your worth and inner power to be able to walk away rather than remain stuck and settling for less.

It may be worth remembering at this point what we touched on in Chapter 3: that people will fall away as you embark on a self-discovery and spiritual journey – it is a sad but unavoidable truth. As you change and grow and evolve, you will no longer resonate with certain people or find a lot in common with them. You changing will trigger reactions in other people, especially those who benefit from you staying the same. It also highlights for others where they are stuck in their lives, so they would rather you stay stuck with them than free yourself and show them how change is possible, especially when they are not ready to see that. And so, if you find people leaving your life, mourn the loss, but please don't use it as an excuse to shrink back to less of yourself. Them leaving will create the space for new people to come in who are aligned with who you are becoming and will meet you as the Goddess that you are.

Reclamation ritual

I would love you to take a moment here to reflect on how you have changed through this journey so far, how perhaps you are not the same as you were a few weeks or months ago and how you may now want, need and desire something different from your life. Maybe you no longer want to settle for what you have been settling for or allowing what you have been allowing or doing what you've been doing. Get honest here about what you need to change in your life. This doesn't mean that you need to make all these changes all at once, but being honest about what isn't working is your brave first step.

Now look at what your part to play may be in these things and what changes you can begin to make as you continue along the Goddess Path.

The Truth About Your Sabotages

Now is also the time to get honest with yourself about the ways in which you self-sabotage and hold yourself back, and therefore don't allow yourself to grow fully into the Goddess that you are. Self-sabotage is when we consciously or unconsciously do (or don't do) things that prevent us from achieving success, happiness, love and purpose. This usually stems from a fear of success, lack of self-worth, imposter syndrome, worrying too much about what others may think or say, or trying to avoid difficult emotions or pain. Just like our shadows, our sabotage tendencies can be sneaky – so sneaky, in fact, that we may not even notice them happening until we realise that the same patterns are repeating in our lives over and over again.

It may be that you were late in applying for the promotion as you feared that you wouldn't be good enough for the role anyway, or that it would mean accepting new responsibility and having to rise above your colleagues or let yourself be seen more. You may want a new relationship, but, deep down, fear being vulnerable or getting hurt or being abandoned so you find constant red flags that aren't there or choose people who will keep playing out your relationship stories and dramas. As you do this, you create a self-fulfilling prophecy and get to keep telling yourself the story that relationships don't work or there are no good partners out there.

Or, my personal favourite is procrastination, and I am absolutely brilliant at this. Every book I've ever written I've left right to the deadline, including this one. I may tell you that it's because I work better under pressure, and there is some truth in that. But between you and me, if I'm honest, it's because there is a part of me that's terrified of letting you all down and not writing a good enough book to help you in the way I really want to.

Reclamation ritual

Lunar work can be so powerful in seeing our self-sabotaging patterns of behaviours. At the new moon, the beginning of a brand-new lunar cycle, set intentions for what you want to achieve, create and manifest in your life over the next month. Over the next two weeks, as the moon waxes and grows bigger and brighter in the sky, this is the outward phase of the lunar cycle where, just like the moon, you let yourself be seen, shine and put yourself out there, doing all you can to make your new moon intentions come true. We then get the full moon, who illuminates our lives and shows us what we did achieve and make happen, and where we got in our own way. It's here that you begin to notice that you will come up against the same sabotaging behaviours again and again (perhaps in a slightly different disguise).

Perhaps work with a lunar cycle or two and get honest about what your sabotages are. Where do you say you want something and then behave in a completely different way? Do you decide that you want to start getting up early before the rest of your household to meditate and do your Goddess rituals, and then end up staying up really late so that you are tired and groggy the next morning, and can convince yourself that you are not a morning person and rituals don't work for you? Do you set yourself unrealistic goals or expectations or even always aim too low, find yourself always making excuses, starting tomorrow or waiting until everything is perfect?

Get honest about where you get in your own way and dim your magic, power and having all that you are deserving of. Once you have identified your sabotages, see if you can get to the bottom of where they come from and what they are trying to protect you from. Then look at ways you can begin to make small changes to help you to believe in yourself more and overcome your sabotages.

Knowing Your Truth

We come to an interesting part of the Goddess Path now, the part where you begin to reclaim your personal truth. I want to begin this section by saying that no one knows the absolute truth and all the answers until we go 'back there', back to where our souls came from, if you do indeed believe there is a such a place.

I truly believe that each one of us is a soul having a human experience. I believe that, before we come down to earth, our soul sits with our guides and decides on the lessons, challenges, situations and experiences that we are going to face in this lifetime to help us to learn, grow and evolve. And that we go back at the end of our lives to review this lifetime and decide on our lessons for the next one.

Part of the spiritual and Goddess journey is discovering what your truths are and what feels right and resonates for you. This gets easier the more you get to know yourself and have first-hand life, Goddess and spiritual experiences. It can be very confusing when you begin – there are Goddesses and crystals, reiki and energy healing, lunar magic and astrology, spirit guides and past-life regression, this person saying this is the way and that person saying that is the way, and I know, for me, I wanted to do it all. I flitted between believing one thing and then another and becoming a crystal healer, regression therapist, reiki healer and working with guides and then Goddesses and then oracle cards, to name just a few!

But, over time, you learn what works for you and begin to establish your own inner truths – a set of beliefs that you can build the foundation of your life upon, that make everything in your life easier and more meaningful. You will find your own personal connection with the divine feminine and your inner Goddess. So, if anything that I've said throughout this book hasn't felt right for you, that's not your truth. Take what feels good and leave the rest. Discovering your own truth is part of the journey of the Goddess Path.

I also want to mention here to be careful who you listen to. You wouldn't take relationship advice from your perpetually single friend, or investment advice from someone who was always broke. Everyone who ever gives you advice does so based on their own life and lived experiences and what they believe to be true. This is where finding your own truth becomes valuable as you begin to trust your own knowing more and seek external advice and validation much less.

The more you can establish your beliefs and truth, the more you will be able to stand firm in your Goddess power and inner knowing. When I first started my spiritual journey over 20 years ago, I wanted everyone to know and believe what I knew and believed. It came partly from a well-meaning place, as these things were changing my life so much that I wanted to help others in the same way. But, while we are being truthful, it was because I didn't fully believe in them and so others believing in them somehow made them real and gave me permission to believe in them too. I needed that external validation as my beliefs weren't strong enough.

Now, after walking this path for decades, I know my beliefs and truths in the very core of me. I believe them in every fibre and cell of my being; I feel them as truth in my bones. It wouldn't matter anymore who else believed them – these are my truths, and they are true for me and help me to show up as me and live a happy, purposeful and fulfilled life. I can now be questioned on my beliefs or have others doubt them and I don't crumble. I stand firm in my own truth and knowing.

Reclamation ritual

Take some time here to really feel into what your truths are now that you know yourself and the Goddess in a much deeper way. What is your relationship with the Goddess, what has she taught you? What is your relationship with yourself, what have you learned about yourself? Do you believe in souls, past lives, spirit guides, everything happening for a reason, energy healing, and so on?

Your answers don't have to be concrete or your beliefs forever – these may change as you deepen into your relationship with yourself, your soul and the Goddess, and learn, grow and evolve more along your journey. But for now, start to gently question and explore what you believe or know to be true at this stage along the Goddess Path.

Speaking Your Truth

We hear an awful lot about speaking your truth, but what does that actually mean? To me, it begins with knowing who you are, what you value, what you believe and what you want. It means staying true to who you are and not hiding what you feel for fear of what others may think or say. It's being able to stay true to your opinions, beliefs and needs, and speak openly about them. Speaking your truth means sharing yourself authentically and truthfully from your heart, with no second-guessing, censoring or fear.

As you get to know yourself further, the easier this becomes. As you stay true to you, you no longer need to shrink or hide yourself, and you gain more confidence in being all of yourself. You no longer have to live a lie in any area of your life or agree with things you don't agree with or bend and break yourself to keep the peace; instead, you get to be real and authentic and let all of you shine through.

The more you are brave enough to speak your truth, the more you will be able to communicate your needs and are no longer left feeling disappointed or let down in life. We often have this misconception that people should know what we want and need, especially those who love us, but we can't expect anyone to really know what we need unless we tell them, and speaking your truth helps you to do that. It helps you to take back your power to express yourself fully and authentically and free yourself to be all of you.

Reclamation ritual

Begin by looking at any areas of your life or people around you who you currently don't feel able to speak your truth with, and why. Do you find yourself nodding and agreeing with certain family members about things you just don't agree with? Or never speaking up and sharing your opinion around certain friends? Or holding back your ideas and viewpoints in work meetings? Maybe you don't make your needs known in your relationship as it saves an argument. Then, begin to practise speaking up and speaking out a little at a time. Perhaps begin with people you don't know that well, who have no preconceived opinions about you. The more you speak your truth, the more empowered you will become and the more you will inspire and free others to use the power of their voices too.

INVOKE THE GODDESS

Kali is the Hindu Goddess of change, time, empowerment, destruction, death and rebirth. A raw, wild force of feminine power, she will help you to know yourself, own yourself and free yourself to fearlessly follow your truth.

Kali is the one to have by your side when you know things need to change in your life, and sometimes she knows long before you do and will create upheaval, disruption and chaos to get you to wake up and pay attention.

She is a force to be reckoned with, and you will know when she weaves her wild ecstatic dance into your life, but she is a force of change, liberation, truth and transformation, and your life will never be the same again once you've walked the path with Kali.

Bringing a fierce, protective love, she will help you to slay your sabotages, let go of limiting beliefs, old structures and old habits that keep you stuck in your comfort zone and hiding your truth. She will support you in letting any old versions of you die away so that you can be reborn into more of your fullness, truth and presence, and allow the full feminine life force to flow through you.

She will demand that you stop hiding from yourself and hiding your full self from others, and claim your fullest expression, discovering and awakening to your inner truth and finding the courage to fearlessly share that with the world.

Here are some ways to invite the fierce, powerful Kali into your life:

Release what no longer serves you

Hold a releasing ceremony with Kali where you get honest about what you need to change, transform and let go of in your life. This may be relationships, your job or a version of you that is afraid or sabotages. Perhaps write it down, speak it all out loud to Kali and then safely burn the paper, feeling Kali's fire of transformation take it. This doesn't necessarily mean you have to make all the changes straight away, but even speaking your truth out loud and having it witnessed by Kali will be so empowering. If you're ready, ask her to assist you in making these changes, and let the transformation commence.

Let Kali speak through you

If you are afraid to begin speaking your truth, ask Kali to speak through you. She will help you to find your voice and the courage to begin to use it, especially the more you speak your truth to her. Tell Kali of your sabotages, your deepest darkest fears and what you know and believe within you to be true. Let her be the witness of you beginning the process of baring your soul. Tell her everything you fear to tell anyone else just yet and let her help you to find, trust and know the truth of your being. Then, when it's time to share your voice with the world, channel your inner Kali and hear her roar.

Ecstatically dance your truth

Kali is often depicted in a wild, frenzied ecstatic dance, usually on top of Shiva, which represents her having mastery over the process of life through her constant cycles of creation, life and death. Find mastery over your own life in the same way. Pick some music, play it loud and invite Kali in to dance with you. Dance your truth, your sabotages and what changes you want to make. Connect to the raw, primal core of you and let all your truth be expressed through wild dance and movement. Don't hold anything back – dance your truth and feel it alive within you all the way to your bones.

Embody the Archetypes

The wild woman

Call on your inner wild woman to bring you the courage to be all of you and stand in your truth. Whenever you feel yourself shrinking, feel your inner wild woman hold you in your truth.

The visionary

Let your inner visionary help you to explore, uncover and connect to your innermost truth, and then begin to create the world around you from that. She will help you to clearly see your truth and create any necessary change to manifest your vision.

Live Your Truth

Try living in your total truth for a full day. Live by your beliefs, values and be radically honest with yourself in every moment of the day about every thought, word and action you take. Try to only speak the truth all day and really own yourself and your truth.

AFFIRMATIONS TO RECLAIM YOUR TRUTH

O   'I embrace change.'

O   'It is safe to express my truth.'

O   'I live an authentic life.'

O   'I am free to be me.'

O   'My inner truth guides me.'

O   'I speak my truth.'

It is my hope that you can now stand clear in your truth and authenticity, and begin to share more of you with the world. From this place of knowing yourself, let's now look at how you can reclaim rest and receiving.

'It's time to start to slow down and listen my Love, and, in doing so, reclaim rest and receiving, for this is where you'll truly begin to find and know the Goddess within.'

Chapter 10

RECLAIM REST AND RECEIVING

We live in a world that tells us that our worth is equated to how much we are doing, leading us to live lives where we are constantly pushing, struggling, striving and somehow trying to prove ourselves. We have been led to believe that being busy is a sign of success, but if we want to truly know and embody the feminine, we need to break that illusion.

The masculine is 'doing' energy; the feminine is 'being' and receiving. We can't know the Goddess while we are constantly rushing around and tying ourselves in knots. When we are constantly on the go, rushing here, there and everywhere, and filling every waking moment with doing something, we lose touch not only with the deep inner feminine voice of the Goddess, but also with ourselves. It's time to start to slow down and listen my Love, and, in doing so, reclaim rest and receiving, for this is where you'll truly begin to find and know the Goddess within.

Resigning from the perpetual state of being busy and disconnected from your inner world and reclaiming and embracing slow living, flow and time for deep inner listening is a radical act of self-love. This is the beginning of a beautiful journey back to knowing yourself and the Goddess within.

Reclaim Rest

So many of us struggle to rest, finding the voice in our heads telling us we should be doing something at all times or jumping up off the sofa when we hear someone come home for fear they will catch us resting and judge us as being lazy. We somehow feel that we need to 'earn' rest and are only allowed it when we have reached the point of utter exhaustion, but even then can never fully allow ourselves to relax and let go. We see resting as such a sign of weakness and push so hard against our emotional and hormonal fluctuations and changing energy levels, trying to prove that we can keep going and do it all but, in doing so, we end up doing less. We ignore burnout signals from our body and soul until it hits us so hard, we end up on the floor.

This is where regular rest is so powerful, transformative and life-changing as you take time to recharge your Goddess energies. You wouldn't dream of going on a long journey with an empty petrol tank or heading out for a big day with a low mobile phone battery. Yet we do this to ourselves on a regular basis, continuing to push ourselves out there into the world when we have nothing left to give.

Reclamation ritual

If you want to truly reclaim the Goddess within, it begins with reclaiming regular rest. One of the easiest ways to begin to do this is to start to honour either your own cycle or the moon's. The days of the dark/new moon and the days of your bleed are the lowest emotional and energetic points of the cycle, and give us a permission slip to rest and withdraw from the world into ourselves.

Our ancestors would have gathered in the red tent during the days of the new moon/their bleed to honour, nurture and nourish themselves and give themselves what they needed (we'll cover more of this in the next chapter). It's time to reclaim the red tent and allow yourself deep and regular rest and rejuvenation.

Begin to mark out a few hours, an evening, a day – whatever you can manage around this time – to indulge in guilt-free rest and self-care. I promise you that you giving yourself this time to rest will make you a better mother, friend, daughter, sister and all-round Goddess through the rest of the month.

Take some time too to consider your relationship with rest. Do you feel it's lazy, weak or unnecessary? Where did those stories come from? Did you witness your mother never sitting down and always self-sacrificing or do you hear the voice of someone else in your head telling you that you 'should be doing something' each time you try to rest?

Over the coming weeks, reclaim rest by allowing yourself to do things you'd never normally let yourself do. Maybe you get under the duvet or run a bubble bath in the middle of the day, get into bed at 8pm with a book and a hot water bottle, or spend an entire Sunday moving slowly and not getting dressed. Listen to your body and what she is asking for and offer yourself the gift of some deep, true rest. Your inner Goddess will not only thank you for it, she'll also thrive from it.

Self-Care Is Not Selfish

While we are talking of rest and nurturing and nourishing your-self, I want to add a little reminder here that self-care is not selfish. In fact, it's the opposite and it's necessary if you want to be able to show up in the world as the Goddess that you truly are. It's impos-sible to be your brightest, shiniest, most powerful, intuitive Goddess self when you are depleted, exhausted and burned out.

Somewhere along the way, especially as women, we got told that being a good person means being selfless and putting every-one else's needs above our own. But I would go as far as to argue that, doing that, is in fact selfish as you deplete yourself and your energy over time and subconsciously tell yourself that you and your needs don't matter as much as those of others. In doing so, you dim yourself and your Goddess.

I'm not for a moment saying don't show up for or take care of anyone else, but they tell you to put your own oxygen mask on first for a reason. You cannot take care of or help anyone else when you have an empty tank and nothing at all to give.

If you tell yourself that you have no time for self-care this is when you need it the most. This is a sure-fire sign that you are on the treadmill towards burnout and have lost touch with the God-dess within. Another little reminder here – you do not need to earn self-care. Part of embracing the Goddess Path is loving and hon-ouring yourself enough to want to take care of yourself in the best way possible.

Reclamation ritual

Self-care is knowing what you need in each moment and giving that to yourself. It's showing up for yourself and making you and your needs important. So, for the next week or so, make your needs a priority. Each morning, check in with your body, your heart and the Goddess within, and ask yourself what you need that day and aim to give that to yourself. It may be that you feel tired and need an early night or to speak a truth, set a boundary or just allow yourself more time for fun and flow through the day.

Self-care can be massages, bubble baths and face masks. It can also be knowing when to put yourself to bed to ensure that you get enough sleep and eating your greens and getting your five a day. It can be meditation, breathwork, weightlifting and yoga. It's also knowing when you've taken on too much and saying no, setting boundaries, holding yourself accountable to promises you make yourself and not letting yourself talk horribly to yourself, especially when you are tired and run down.

Slow Down to Know Yourself

When you are constantly rushing, busy and immersed in the noise of the outside world, it's virtually impossible to hear the voice of your deep inner wisdom, your intuition and Goddess guidance. But very often we rush and run for this exact reason, so that we can try to avoid the niggling voice within that's telling us that we are in the wrong relationship or job or need to make certain changes in our lives. When we are 'too busy' to listen or do anything about it, we can pretend not to know about the ways in which we are living out of alignment, abandoning ourselves or ignoring the Goddess within.

The answers we are looking for will not be found out there in the noise of the world, they will be found in the stillness and silence within. This is where the Goddess will speak to us and through us. It's only by allowing yourself to slow down that you will catch up with yourself enough to know yourself and what you truly want and desire. Slowing down is a radical act of self-care and self-love, especially in a world that is vying for your attention and benefits from keeping you distracted and looking to the outside for answers.

Resign from being busy, allow the outside world to rush around you and instead find calm in the chaos. Let your inner world become slow, calm and quiet. Slow down and sink into the feminine wisdom within – that's where you'll find the Goddess and all you seek.

Reclamation ritual

Take some time over the next week or so to notice how much you are always rushing and your life is one big to-do list. Do you ever allow yourself to move slowly through life, enjoying the moment, connected to your inner world and sense of self? Or are you always rushing from home to work, from meeting to meeting, to get things done, walking quickly, multitasking a hundred things at once and missing the world and messages within and around you?

Carve out daily time to slow down and reconnect to your inner world. This may be as simple as taking a minute, placing your hands over your belly and your heart, and taking some long, slow, deep breaths feeling the breath move through your body and dropping your awareness out of your head and into your inner world. The more you can add little pockets of peace into your day, the more you will be able to feel the feminine within.

When you are trying to solve a problem or feel lost, disconnected or uncertain, stop trying to solve it with your mind or grasping the outside world to find something or someone to give you answers – drop into the well of wisdom within you and really be with yourself. Imagine turning the volume dial down on the outside world and letting it all drift away, and go inwards to your truth, your wisdom and your inner knowing. Listen.

Less Doing, More Being

We've been raised in a hustle culture, a 'man's world', with talk of being a 'girl boss' and that the only way to get ahead and be successful is to dedicate yourself to the grind; that to get what you want, you have to work hard or suffer somehow. Even in the workplace, the masculine traits of being competitive, assertive, emotionally detached and racking up 60-plus-hour weeks are celebrated and the feminine qualities of intuition, collaboration, empathy and care carry far less recognition.

Stress is sadly on the rise, with 74 per cent of UK adults saying they have felt so stressed at some point over the last year, they have felt overwhelmed or unable to cope. In the workplace, 79 per cent of people report being stressed, with women suffering 45 per cent more work-related stress than men.[1] I truly believe that this is due to us pushing against the feminine and trying to live up to unrealistic expectations of being 'on' and available all the time, spending too much time in our masculine doing, doing, doing at the expense of our feminine energy. Some of the worst bosses I have ever had have been women, as they have tried to show up in the workplace as men rather than in their true feminine powers.

I remember an old client of mine worked as a lawyer for a big American firm. She was so burned out, stressed and exhausted that she could barely even function anymore. She came to me one day full of relief as her work had agreed that she could go part-time. So happy for her, I asked her what her new hours would be, to which she replied 8am to 4pm. When did 8–4 become part-time?! How have we glorified working and doing so much, leaving no time for being and, more importantly, living? We see stress as a marker of success and always being busy as a badge of honour. But what if we've got it all wrong? What if the true marker of success was being able to work and rush around less and spend more time in nature, resting, napping, with family and friends and doing things that nurtured our souls and filled our hearts with joy?

We will not find more of ourselves or our value and worth in the hustle and grind, living too much in our masculine and keeping our nervous systems frazzled – this is how we lose ourselves and our connection to the feminine. I know this was so true for me when writing this book. On a tight deadline, there would be times when I would sit for hours bashing away at the keyboard telling myself I was too busy and had too much to do to go outside in nature and walk, a daily almost non-negotiable for me. It was only when the writer's block and frustration became too much that I finally gave up the doing and went outside – that was when the magic happened. Surrounded by nature, with my feet on the earth, the sun on my face and the sound of birdsong around me, I would suddenly be hit with inspiration and answers, and parts of the book I'd been struggling with would suddenly write themselves as a stream of consciousness in my mind. I have hundreds of voice notes in my phone of these words just pouring through me, and they did not come in the moments of chaining myself to a desk doing and forcing. They came in the moments of being, of giving up the grind and surrendering to being in the feminine connection and flow.

When we carve out more time to simply be, whatever that may mean for you, this is when we can find true inspiration, answers and access to the divine feminine energy. This is when we start to find ourselves and, rather than living on high alert, our nervous systems can begin to take a deep sigh and relax.

In allowing yourself time to do less, you'll achieve more as you get to fill yourself all the way back up again and have so much more to give from a place of being connected to your true inner well of wisdom, strength, power and magic. It's through rest that you get to become all of who you can be.

Reclamation rituals

Be present

Try taking regular moments through the day where you are not 'doing' anything; you're just allowing yourself to 'be'. This is where you will find the feminine, in presence, being fully immersed in the moment, being in our bodies, hearts and souls, feeling and sensing.

Allow yourself to be fully present in the moment and take it all in. Take in how you're feeling, your surroundings, your breath – fully immerse yourself in the present moment. Notice if any resistance or discomfort comes up or you find yourself wanting to do something or telling yourself you're bored. Now see if you can allow yourself to simply be, here, now. There is no past, no future, just this moment. Let everything in and around you slow all the way down. Be present with yourself and your surroundings, and sink into the presence of just being.

Don't 'do', just 'be'

Find one thing daily that brings you joy and fulfilment and try not to 'do' that thing, but be it. So, you may love to dance and move your body – try not to 'do' the dancing, but become the movement and feel the aliveness and joy that rushes through your body. Perhaps for you it's time in nature, where you let yourself fully immerse in her beauty and energy. Think about it, you can't 'do' nature. Even when we speak about it we tend to say, 'I want to go and "be" in nature.' Nature teaches us how to be, here, now. There is a doing in nature as she blooms and grows and sheds and releases, but it is never rushed or forced, it all happens in perfect timing.

Redefine what success means for you

Are you going to continue to buy into the outdated narrative that success is long working hours, stress, financial achievements and reaching a certain point on the corporate ladder? Instead, create your own measure of success – what would being successful truly mean for you? Would it be to be truly tapped into your intuition and sense of self, to only work three days a week, to have the freedom to work your own hours or take a break each afternoon to walk in nature? Would being successful mean a sense of inner harmony and happiness, more time to dedicate to rituals, a sense of purpose or spending quality time with family and friends who love you? What would being successful truly mean to you?

Open Yourself to Receive

Very often we say that we want something in our lives, yet when we are always busy, always rushing, always switched on, there is no room to be able to receive it. The Goddess teaches us how to receive.

Especially as women, I often find we struggle to truly receive. With many of us recovering people-pleasers, fixers, givers and the ones who take care of everyone else, we feel the burden of having to do it all, yet struggle to accept or ask for help. Our ability to receive is also equated to our levels of self-worth and whether we believe ourselves to be deserving of receiving what we want.

One way that we block the receiving flow is by not having the space for what we truly want in our lives. You may say that you want a deep, committed, romantic relationship, but then you are out every single night, busy every moment of the day and your diary is chock-a-block. Where would that relationship fit into your life? Is there really any room for a committed relationship? Do you have the energy for it, the time for it, the space for it? We must create the room to receive what we want in our lives.

We do the same thing when we seek answers, guidance and wisdom from the Goddess and/or the universe. We ask for a sign or a message, but then we don't allow ourselves to receive it as we are too busy pushing our own agendas as we believe that little human us knows best. I often smile to myself about how little human me believes she knows better than the entire universe!

Human us often only dreams small for fear that we won't achieve what we want. We will try to grip, manipulate and hold on to the way that we want it to be when our Goddess selves know all that we are capable of, and the universe is like, 'If you'd just let go of what you're holding on to, I have all of this to give to you and it's even better than you ever imagined.' Now, whenever I am man-ifesting or asking for anything from the universe, I always ask 'for this or something better' as that creates the space for me to receive whatever is best for my own highest good.

When our hands are full, there is nowhere for us to be able to receive the gifts that want to make their way to us. So, practise letting go of expectations and instead being open to receiving all the goodness that wants to make its way to you. The more we open ourselves up to receive, and through this journey know what we are worthy and deserving of, the more the Goddess can weave her magic through our lives.

Reclamation ritual

Practise receiving this week. Notice what you do when someone tries to give you something, even as small as buying you a cup of coffee. Do you straight away try to give something back? When someone asks if you're ok, do you say, 'Fine, how are you?' and turn it back to hearing all about them? When someone compliments you, do you reply with, 'Oh this old thing'? Can you ask for or receive help, or do you struggle through all alone (and then often feel resentful that no one ever helps you or cares about how you are)?

This week, if someone gives you something, just say thank you and receive it fully. Receive compliments, receive any offers of help or someone letting you out in a queue, or a hug or a kind word. Notice that the more you receive, the more comes to you.

There is a beautiful song by Fia called 'Receive' which I often play, especially when I notice I am struggling against my feminine flow and trying to do and push and force. It often helps me, too, when I feel afraid and unsure and as though nothing is working or flowing. The answer in times like this is very often not in more doing – which actually blocks the flow of all that wants to come to me; it's in receiving.

To do this, try playing this song, or another that resonates more with you. Lie on the floor and feel yourself sink deep into the arms and support of Mother Earth and allow yourself to receive. Feel the creative feminine energy flowing through you, your birth right. Breathe here and let yourself simply receive all that is wanting to make its way to you.

Another beautiful ritual that I love to add into my day is throwing my arms and heart wide open and saying out loud, 'I am open to receiving all the love, luck and abundance in the world.' You may change the words if there is something that you would rather be open to receiving, but let the Goddess know that you are truly ready and just wait and see what she brings your way.

Soften and Surrender to the Flow

The Goddess teaches us how to soften and surrender to what is and to trust in the flow of life. So often our minds want to try to have it all figured out and to have guarantees. We end up doing mental gymnastics trying to micromanage, grip, hold and control parts of our lives, either trying to force an outcome or hold on to something that's not meant to be held on to anymore.

But this is the masculine way. The masculine energy wants to fix and solve and figure it out, which is wonderful in the moment and is needed to solve a problem. However, it's exhausting when we spend most of our time doing, fixing and controlling. This is where we need to learn to soften into the feminine, who teaches us to trust and surrender and go with the flow. When we begin to trust in the Goddess and ourselves, we can begin to flow with life rather than force. We can soften into what is, trusting that, even if we don't know the exact outcome yet or how it is all going to figure itself out, we trust in the Goddess, the universe and, most of all, ourselves enough to know that, no matter what happens, we can face it and will get through it.

Everything that happens in your life is intended to give you the necessary lessons, challenges, insights and experiences that your soul needs to grow, evolve and expand, and take the journey that you chose for you this lifetime. This one belief has got me through so much in my own life – that my soul has chosen this for me, and my soul wouldn't choose anything that I couldn't get through. Whenever I am going through something particularly challenging or difficult, I remind myself of this and it shifts my entire perspective and helps me to remain connected to a higher source of power and wisdom.

When we can begin to trust and believe that we are always being supported and guided and that our souls have chosen every experience for us, the more magical, purposeful and in flow our lives become. Your soul wouldn't choose anything that you couldn't get through. You came here with a unique soul story that your soul wants to live out through you, and that the Goddess wants to animate and bring to life through you. The more you can begin to surrender into trust, ease and grace, the more the feminine energies can work their creative magic through you and guide you to where you need to be.

When we push against the flow and swim against the tide, the harder and more exhausting life gets. So, instead, surrender into the arms of the divine feminine and let her hold and carry you to where you need to be. Find a deep enough trust in yourself (or initially the Goddess as she will lend you her support until you find the same levels of trust in yourself) to be in the space of the unknown, knowing that this is where the magic happens. Let go of the sides, stop gripping and trying to control, and let yourself be carried, held and supported.

Reclamation ritual

Learn to sit in the space of surrender and deep trust without trying to have it all figured out. Notice when you're in doing and fixing mode, and instead see if you can let go, surrender and trust. In any moments when it does all feel too much, call on the Goddess for guidance and support – 'I'm not sure what to do right now, please help me' – and allow her support, wisdom and guidance to flow into your life.

INVOKE THE GODDESS

Both the Roman Goddess **Venus** and her Greek sister, **Aphrodite**, are the Goddesses of love, beauty, fertility, prosperity and desire, and teach us the art of self-nurturing, self-love, rest, receiving and inner harmony.

These Goddesses show us that much of our true feminine power is activated and found in our softness and the embodiment of feminine energy which, alongside being wild and sometimes fierce, is slow, sensual, pleasurable and peaceful, and doesn't like to be rushed.

These Goddesses fully welcome being worshipped and adored and as such will teach you how to slow down, self-worship and truly allow yourself to rest in the joy and pleasure of your own existence, rather than always trying to prove and rush your way through life and missing the

moment. Whichever of these sister Goddesses you resonate with the most, both will guide you on an inner journey
of self-discovery and finding yourself in softness, surrender
and taking care of yourself first and foremost.

They will teach you how to revel in and enjoy
moments of pure unadulterated rest and receiving, and
to find satisfaction and contentment in moments of
'doing' nothing yet 'being' utterly present and luxuriating
in the feminine energies of bliss and pleasure.

Look at Venus in your birth chart

Venus also has a planet named after her. A planet that
can only be seen at certain times of the day and night as
she switches between a morning and evening star, taking
regular rest from our skies and disappearing all together
for around 50 days at a time.

Venus in your birth chart teaches you about your
values and shows you how best to care for yourself, how
you receive and where you find your worth. She will teach
you more about your desires, pleasures and indulgences,
and how you can invite more harmony into your life.

Look at what your Venus sign is (you can get a free birth
chart on my website: kirstygallagher.com) and then come
up with some ways in which you can nurture and take care
of your Venus placement and receive her gifts and lessons.

Harness feminine Fridays

Friday is ruled by Venus, making it the ideal day to dedicate to slowing down and being present with the

Goddess. You may allow yourself a slower morning on a Friday, a day free of meetings or outside demands on your energy and time, if possible, or the promise of a long bubble bath or early night at the end of the day.

This doesn't need to be weekly, or even all day, but the more you can carve out regular times for rest and self-honouring, the more you will benefit from these practices and notice a big difference in how you can show up the other six days of the week.

If nothing else, make Fridays a day of the Goddess and remember to go gently and slowly through your day, pausing and being present as often as you can. Notice if you're rushing, juggling or pushing, and ask the Goddess to help you to reconnect back to inner presence and peace, and to rest in the Goddess within.

Use rose quartz

Rose quartz is not only the crystal of self-love, self-care and self-worth, it is also the crystal of the divine feminine energy. Sometimes known as the Venus stone, it is also associated with Aphrodite as legend says that when she was rushing to save her lover Adonis, she cut herself on a briar bush and their blood seeped into the ground to stain the quartz pink.

Carry a piece of rose quartz with you – you could even wear it as jewellery – or keep a piece on your desk at work or somewhere in your home. Each time you look at it or find yourself holding it, use this as a reminder to slow down and rest in your feminine energy for just a few moments – this could be three to five deep breaths.

Anytime you notice yourself rushing through life, hold your rose quartz, connect to the energy of Venus or Aphrodite and feel their energy embrace you, encouraging you to be and receive.

Give yourself a rest permission slip

Write yourself a love letter from Venus or Aphrodite of all the ways in which you deserve to give yourself regular rest. This is a permission slip from her to worship yourself. You don't need to earn rest, but you do deserve it, and this is a beautiful way of you giving yourself permission if you struggle with people-pleasing, putting others first, setting boundaries around your time and energy or if you simply struggle to allow yourself to rest. See this as an instruction from the Goddess to take you further along the Goddess Path and to receive her wisdom and guidance, as she writes you rest receipts.

You could also involve family members or friends in this (or staff members or colleagues) by writing each other permission slips to take rest – a few hours on the sofa to enjoy a TV show, an early night, uninterrupted time in the garden or bath or in nature, a day off or to not have to fix, please or be responsible for anyone else for a few hours. Become the divine feminine embodiment by ensuring that people stick to these permission slips without feeling guilty or making excuses (and make sure that you do the same for yourself).

Embody the Archetypes

The mother

Call on your inner mother and sink into her warm embrace. Feel her whisper to you that it's ok to rest. Receive her love and support, and let her hold you and show you the beauty in slowing down.

The priestess

Let your inner priestess show you how much more can be achieved by worship, devotion and intention rather than rushing, forcing and pushing. Begin to live from a place of connection to the feminine, and make slowing down to receive her a priority.

Worship Your Own Altar

In the same way that you are learning to worship the Goddesses in these pages, worship yourself, your energy and time in the same way. Self-worship by giving yourself regular time to rest, receive and be present with your inner Goddess. When you notice yourself depleted, stressed or running on empty, worship your own altar (of your body, mind, heart and soul). Ideally, don't wait until it gets to that point and carve out time, even a few moments a day, to receive rest and divine feminine energies.

AFFIRMATIONS TO RECLAIM REST AND RECEIVING

○ 'Self-care is not selfish.'
○ 'I give myself full permission to rest/receive/slow down.'
○ 'I embrace slow living.'
○ 'To me, true success means [insert your definition of true success].'
○ 'I surrender to the Goddess flow.'
○ 'It is safe to slow down.'
○ 'I am open to receive.'

You've now embraced rest and receiving, and, in doing so, I hope that you have reclaimed and welcomed in even more of the feminine energies. Let's take this new-found connection to the Goddess and use it to reclaim your seasons and cycles.

'It's time to reclaim our seasons and cycles and, in doing so, reclaim the Goddess and part of ourselves.'

Chapter 11

RECLAIM SEASONS AND CYCLES

Women are cyclical beings. Since the dawn of time, we have moved in rhythm with nature, the moon and the seasons. Just like nature and the moon, women have a natural cycle, an inner rhythm, not only in our menstrual cycles, but also in the transitional phases that we move through on our life journey. Yet, over time, we have been taught to deny and push against this. We worry that today we feel differently to yesterday, get shamed for our shifting emotions and force ourselves to keep going in the times our bodies and souls are crying out for rest. And, as we do this, we silence the Goddess and ignore the wisdom of our bodies, losing contact with the immense amount of feminine wisdom, power and magic within.

Your needs differ in each phase of your cycle and each season of your life, and the more you can begin to honour and understand that, the more you'll honour and understand the Goddess, and yourself.

As you move through this chapter, you will see that your own natural cycles and those of the moon, nature and the Goddess cannot be separated; they are all one and the same – because rhythms, cycles, seasons are encoded in our blood, our bones, our

DNA. It's time to reclaim these cycles and, in doing so, reclaim the Goddess and part of ourselves.

The Triple Goddess:
The Maiden, Mother and Crone

We touched upon some of these feminine archetypes in Chapter 1, but let's look at them now as to how they relate to the natural seasons and cycles of a woman's journey through her own life.

The triple Goddess – maiden, mother, crone – represents a woman's journey through menarche (the first bleed), menstruation, childbirth and menopause. These are hugely transitional times in a woman's life journey and there was a time when rituals were held to celebrate these milestones. There is an ancient Native American saying which sums this up perfectly: 'At her first bleeding, a woman meets her power. During her bleeding years, she practices it. At menopause, she becomes it.'

These archetypes once again mirror the seasons of nature and the phases of the moon, and, just as each season in nature or each phase of the moon offers different energy, lessons and insights, the same applies to these transitional stages of a woman's life.

Lately, as we are now living longer and choosing to have children later, new categories have been added to this list: mage, which are the years from perimenopause into menopause before you reach crone; and enchantress, which is when you are no longer a maiden, but haven't become a mother – we'll explore these below too.

It's important to remember that some women may not follow this natural cycle, with not all women getting married or having children, but we will all experience the energy of each of these archetypes in our lives. We will also embody and experience the energy of each of these archetypes through our menstrual cycles (more on that below) and can work with these energies in that way.

The maiden

Said to encompass the first 25 years of a women's life, her true transition into maiden energy comes with her menarche. This is the phase of our lives when we are going through many changes in our bodies, hormones and emotions as we develop and grow into womanhood. With typically no ties, no children and no big responsibilities, this is our time of freedom, fun and liberation as we explore who we are and begin to seek our place in the world.

These youthful years tend to be filled with optimism about the future, discoveries, independence and rebellion. The maiden is filled with energy, passion for life and wants to adventure and explore as much as she can. With the increase in social media and media-fuelled celebrity beauty standards, however, this can nowadays be a time filled with comparison, anxiety and trying to achieve unrealistic expectations in lifestyle, looks and achievements. That's why it's important for women to walk the Goddess Path from early on in life, so that we claim our own sense of self-worth and know who we are from a young age. Meditation, mindfulness and inner work are important for the maiden to find an inner anchor to cope with the external pressures of the modern-day world.

If you have maidens in your life, teach them about the Goddess Path and the importance of self-belief, self-knowing and self-awareness young; help them to know they are already enough as they are.

The mother

Between the ages of 25 and 45, this is the phase of life when a woman is in full bloom and likely her most fertile, whether you have children or not. Those of us who have children will go through the huge initiation process of birth and raising a child/ren. Those of us who don't may use these years to birth a business, career, projects, ideas or anything else that wants to be birthed through you.

These are years of accepting big life responsibilities and devoting our energies to the creation of life, whether that be children or dreams, desires and ideas. We are deeply connected to feminine life force energy and our own inner strength and ability to create, nurture, provide and protect.

Remember to mother yourself during this phase too, as this transitionary time can leave many women struggling once more with outside expectations and the big life changes this phase brings. Women with children can struggle with an initial loss of personal identity and having to manage it all alone, and it's important at this stage, just like the saying goes, to find your village and lean on the support around you. Women unable or choosing not to have children suffer the constant questions and judgement from the outside world, and this comes with its own set of challenges. That's why it's so important to have a strong self-care practice and to call on your inner mother to hold, protect and take care of you.

If you have mothers in your life, offer them support and encouragement and let them know they don't need to do it alone. If you have mothers without children in your life, support them in birthing their projects, hopes and dreams.

The crone

The original crone years were over the age of 45, but back then we didn't live as long and tended to have children much younger, and so nowadays new categories (see below) have been added and the crone years may be later.

I personally see menopause as being a reclamation of the crone and love everything about women taking this energy back, especially as once women reach a certain age, they are dismissed by our modern society. Deemed as 'past it' and no longer seen as useful, it can be a time when many women feel unappreciated and even invisible. It's time to reclaim the crone energy and see menopause for what it truly is – a transformational rite of passage into deeper wisdom, knowing and Goddess power.

The word 'crone' itself, although now seen as an insult along with hag and witch, originally meant 'old crown' and these women would have been the elders, leaders, healers, medicine women and wise women of their community. When a woman retains her bleed, her 'wise blood', she embodies all the experiences, lessons and wisdom from her life, and can now share this with others from a place of true lived experience and knowing.

It is also usually at this stage of life when women care the least about what society expects and they become less tameable, and I truly believe that's why women in this stage of life have been made to feel so useless by society as a way to keep them down. Crone energy has the power to change the world and we need more women embodying and embracing the power and wisdom that this stage of life brings.

If you have crones in your life, ask questions and make the most of their wisdom. Ask them what they wish they'd done differently, what they cared too much about that they wish they hadn't and what they would do differently, knowing what they now know. Look to them to guide the way forward to changing the world.

The Mage and the Enchantress

The mage – sometimes known as the wild woman, medicine woman or witch – represents the perimenopausal years when women are no longer bearing children but haven't transitioned fully through menopause yet. These are the years after mother, but before you are ready to step into your full crone power.

If you have children, it's likely they are now more self-sufficient and many of the big life responsibilities have eased, meaning that you have more time, freedom and independence to explore who you are and what you now want to do. If you haven't had children, it's likely that you are more established in your career and life.

This is a time of self-discovery and getting to know yourself once again, but now with the immense life wisdom and experience you have gained.

The enchantress represents the years in which you are no longer a maiden, but for whatever reason have not become a mother. You've transitioned from the more innocent maiden phase into a place of more empowerment and self-awareness, and you can now use this to navigate your way through the world.

You are filled with the energy to create and can put this to use in any life areas that you choose – from self-development to adventures, travelling and carving out a career path.

This is a time of wisdom, freedom and self-exploration, and establishing your way in the world, deciding who you want to be and what you want from life.

Menstrual Seasons and Cycles

It is only quite recently that menstrual cycles have been more openly discussed and seen as a tool of empowerment. Sadly, for decades, and for many of you reading this, this wouldn't have been your experience. Menstruation may have held feelings of shame, confusion, secrecy and a sense of it being unclean, impure and something that you don't talk about and just had to suffer through silently. It may have been a subject of ridicule, weakness or embarrassment, and having any slight mood swing blamed on 'having PMT'. In fact, it's been taboo for so long that we've even created names for it to avoid directly referring to what it is: 'the curse', 'the crimson wave', 'the blob', 'Aunt Flo', 'the rag' and other such delightful names.

Did you know that due to strict censorship rules regarding menstrual product advertising, it took until 1985 for the word 'period' to first be used in an advert? Or that it was only in 2017 that menstrual blood was represented by a red liquid, rather than blue?[2]

When and how menstruation became taboo is unclear, but menstrual taboo has succeeded in labelling women somehow inferior beings and used to control, restrict and suppress women over the ages. Could it have been the immense amount of power that women hold during this sacred time of the month that caused the rumours that menstruating women controlled the moon, had dangerous supernatural powers and that women are dirty, impure and sinful while they are bleeding; rumours which caused the tide to turn on how menstruation was viewed?

It hasn't always been this way. Ancient hunter-gatherer societies and historic cultures considered menstruation to be a healing, protective and sacred time, and believed that a menstruating woman had access to higher spiritual powers, psychic abilities and an ability to access deeper wisdom, guidance and intuition. In ancient Greece and Egypt, menstrual blood was thought to hold magical powers and was ingested to increase spiritual power and spread on fields to increase the fertility of the land. In other cultures, women gathered together for a few days at a new moon to menstruate in a moon lodge, menstrual house or red tent. This would have been a sacred time of withdrawal from day-to-day duties and life when women would share, support and encourage each other, and tune more deeply into their heightened inner understanding and intuition. For example, women from the Yurok tribes would go on strike for their moontime, taking time in seclusion to access their powers and meditate on the purpose of their life. They would communally bathe and perform rituals, and bleed alongside the moon. This was the same for the Ojibwe women, who considered menstruation a time of cleaning, renewal and celebrating womanhood. Women would use their time in the moon lodge to rest, cleanse and regather their energies. They would refrain from all other duties and be taken care of by the rest of the tribe.

A woman's ability to bleed without dying was seen as a magical superpower and her blood was seen as a sacred elixir. There is even an ancient Hopi prophecy that says, 'When the women give their blood back to the earth, men will come home from war and the earth shall find peace.'

It's time to reclaim the power of your period, and it's never too late to do that. Start now and take back the wisdom of your sacred moon time.

Reclaiming Your Menstrual Cycle

Our menstrual cycle reflects our cyclical nature and gives us the opportunity to fully renew every 29(ish) days. It can be broken down into four individual cycles, during which your energy, emotions, libido and sense of sense will ebb and flow. When you can begin to track, understand and embrace this for yourself, you take back control of your own life and the power of the feminine life force that moves through you each month. No longer are you tied to the conditioning that life should be the same all day every day, and that we should be the same all day every day; because this is just not the way that life is, especially for us women. As you learn to honour and embrace the fluctuations of your moods, body and tolerance levels, and honour your own natural rhythms, you will learn to harness the power and wisdom of the Goddess within you.

As well as each phase of your menstrual cycle bringing unique gifts and energies, each phase is also associated with a phase of the lunar cycle, a season in nature and one of the feminine archetypes mentioned above. The more you can honour yourself through each one of these phases, the more you will connect to your inner Goddess and your power, wisdom, creative life force and the ability to listen to the voice of your heart, soul and deep intuition.

Before we continue, a quick note: your cycle, just like you, is unique and you may have a longer, shorter or irregular cycle. Your cycle will also change over time depending on what you are going through in your life. You may experience different phases of your cycle in a different way, especially at different times of your life, and that is the point – getting to know and honour your own inner feminine and how she needs to flow.

As you begin to pay attention to and get to know your own cycle, you'll get to know yourself and build a deep relationship with your body and inner rhythm, learning to give yourself what you need when you need it. This is what it truly means to walk the Goddess Path and honour your Goddess within.

I have spoken to several women recently who feel an immense amount of grief and sadness that they were never taught the magic, power and wisdom of their bleed. If you have been through menopause, please first allow yourself a moment to grieve that this wisdom was kept from you. But please know that you can reclaim it by following the cycle of the moon. She will give you a natural cycle that you can still follow and embrace. Mothers, please teach this to your daughters (and sons) so that we can raise a next generation of women who embody their deep feminine wisdom.

Let's look now at ways to embrace your inner seasons and connect to your inner feminine archetypes as you move through each season of your cycle.

Menstruation

Associated with the dark moon phase, winter and the crone/wise woman archetype.

The beginning of your bleed counts as day one, with menstruation usually lasting three to five days. Here oestrogen and progesterone levels drop, and your body begins shedding the uterine lining that was created in your previous cycle.

During this phase, there may be a feeling of exhaustion, vulnerability, tenderness, aching and deep emotion. This is a time for stillness and withdrawal, rest and self-care, and being able to access your deep inner wisdom and intuition.

Work with your crone/wise woman energy by . . .

Going inwards to listen to the wisdom within: Take time for conscious inner listening and let your crone/wise woman speak. Imagine she has a voice, what would she say to you? You may journal as your inner crone and let her impart messages and wisdom that she wishes to share with you. Call on her wisdom for anything you are struggling with; ask her a question and then sit in stillness and let the answers rise from within you.

Setting personal intentions for the month ahead: Journal on your dreams and visions – what you truly want and need – and set yourself some intentions for the month ahead. What will you make happen over the next month? How will you honour yourself and your seasons and cycles more? What will you put your precious energy and focus into?

Honour your inner winter/dark moon energy by . . .

Withdrawing from the world as much as you can: Think of the stillness of nature in the winter as everything withdraws inwards. Think of the few days of the month that the moon withdraws from the sky. In the same way, this is a time to invite stillness into your life to honour your bleed and this time of inner wisdom. If it's possible to have a day off, do so, or at least move through your days as quietly as you can and try to keep your evenings free. Honour this time of deep stillness and withdrawal and allow yourself to rest and receive. This is not a time to give to others, but to focus on yourself.

Consciously releasing all that you no longer need: Just like the cycles of the moon and nature, we get to experience death and

219

rebirth every month through our menstrual cycle. This is the death part of the cycle where we get to use the symbolism of our bleed to shed all that we no longer need.

In a similar way to the dark moon phase of the lunar cycle, the days running up to our period and PMT show us what we don't want and what is out of alignment in our lives. It's usually in these days that emotions we have suppressed come to the surface and we are deep in our feels. Pay attention to your emotions around this time, and what they are showing you around what you need to shed from your life.

Visualise through your bleed that you are shedding and releasing all that's no longer needed. You may take this a step further by offering your blood to the earth or water asking them to help you to cleanse and release all you no longer need.

Follicular phase

Associated with the waxing moon phase, spring and the maiden archetype.

This is the pre-ovulation phase of your cycle which begins on the first day of your period and lasts approximately 14 days (there is some overlap with the menstrual phase, so instead some class this phase as days 6–14). During this phase, your pituitary gland releases a follicle stimulating hormone, and oestrogen levels begin to rise.

This phase brings a sense of rebirth, increased energy levels and a desire to re-emerge and get back out there in the world. Now is the time to take on new projects, move things forward and face challenges. You'll be bursting with creativity, ideas and inspiration.

Work with your maiden energy by . . .

Committing to more play, fun and flirting: Say yes, socialise and take your inner maiden out to play. Allow yourself some time over the next few days to be more carefree, playful and enjoy the moment. Flirt with the coffee barista, the stranger on the street and with life itself; let yourself enjoy the delicious energy of your own beauty and sensuality.

Becoming a manifesting magnet: Look at the intentions you set yourself during your bleed. What can you now do to make these things happen and attract them into your life? Put your energy and focus on what you want and feel your inner maiden dancing within, making you magnetic to what you desire.

Honour your inner spring/waning moon energy by . . .

Setting your creativity free: You may draw, dance, paint, sing – and it doesn't even need to be any good. This is just a time to unleash your creative side and let it begin to flow through you. Watch where you are blocking the flow of creative energy by needing it to be 'perfect' and just have fun.

Growing something: Put your energy, focus, time and attention into growing something, whether that's a new project or idea, a plant or growing a part of yourself, such as letting yourself be seen more or using your voice to speak up for yourself.

Ovulation

Associated with the full moon phase, summer and the mother archetype.

Days 14–21 are your most fertile as your hormones now reach their highest levels. High levels of oestrogen trigger the pituitary gland to produce luteinising hormone, causing an egg to be released from your ovary into the fallopian tube, where it will survive for up to 24 hours.

This is likely to be your happy time of the month and when you feel in your full power, presence and energy. This is the time in your cycle when you'll come into full bloom, so plan big social events or times you need to shine around these days.

Work with your mother energy by . . .

Taking on the world: Let your mother energy help you to multitask, juggle and get things done. Tick off the to-do list, take care of the admin and get things organised, especially things that will support you in being able to slow down in the next phase of your cycle. This is the best time in your cycle to ask for what you want, so let your needs be known.

Being the caregiver: You'll have the energy and inclination to take care of and look after others at this time of your cycle, so use it. Let your inner mother nurture, support and show up for others, taking care of their needs and letting your maternal energy flow.

Honour your inner summer/full moon energy by . . .

Celebrating you: This is the time of the month when you'll likely feel the best about yourself, so celebrate all of who you are. Take yourself shopping, dance in front of the mirror, tell yourself everything you love about yourself and let yourself shine.

Harnessing your sexual energy: Your libido and sexual energy will be at its peak here. This energy, which can create new life, with this being your most fertile time of the month, can also be channelled into creating a new project or something you want to bring into the world. Feel this life force energy within you and put it into what you want to create.

Luteal phase

Associated with the waning moon phase, autumn and the mage/wild woman archetype.

Once the egg has been released, your body begins to produce progesterone to help prepare the lining of the uterus for possible pregnancy. If this doesn't happen, after a week or so oestrogen and progesterone levels will begin to drop, so that the uterus lining begins to break down, which will become your bleed.

Days 22–29 start your journey back inwards towards yourself and beginning to gradually slow down and honour yourself as you get closer to your bleed. This is a time of being in touch with your inner world, reflection, gathering what you need and completion.

Work with your mage/wild woman energy by ...

Expressing your emotions: The more we reject and suppress our emotions and disown our needs, the more likely they are to show up during the premenstrual part of our cycle as more intense PMT symptoms. Put on some loud music and set your wild woman free to stamp, cry, laugh, rage and express how you're feeling.

Setting boundaries: If you've been over-giving, self-abandoning or not honouring your own needs, now is the time to reclaim your time, energy and self. Call on your inner wild woman to help you to put yourself first and free you from boundary fears so that you can honour your waning energy.

Honour your inner autumn/waning moon energy by . . .

Committing to self-care, self-care, self-care: This is where you choose to honour your body's needs and slow down instead of forcing against your natural rhythm – a true act of self-love. The more you can take care of yourself in this phase of your cycle, the more attuned you'll be to yourself and the more you will reap the benefits of this through the rest of your cycle.

Going within: Spend more time in reflection, introspection and inner listening. Pay attention to what's frustrating you and the parts of your life that don't feel in integrity and flow or where you've been self-abandoning and not staying true to you. Journal, meditate, practise yoga and breathwork, and listen to your inner world to hear the truth of what your inner Goddess needs you to know.

Reclamation rituals

Honour your first bleed

Look back to your first period: Do you remember it? Do you remember feeling empowered, scared, ashamed? Or perhaps you have no memory of it at all.

For centuries, traditions all around the world have held rituals to celebrate this sacred rite of passage into womanhood. In many of these ancient practices, these young women were seen to have gained new spiritual powers and were not only celebrated but frequently spent time alone to integrate this power, while receiving visits and wisdom from the older women or crones of the community.

Nowadays, it is becoming much more common to hold an initiation for girls at their menarche, but it's not too late to do this for yourself. Hold a ritual where you meet the 13- or 14-year-old you (or however old you remember or feel you were at your first bleed). Create a safe, sacred space, close your eyes and either imagine yourself back at that time or visualise that younger self version of you with you. Let her share with you how she is feeling, and then hold her and tell her all that you wish she knew back then.

Track your cycles

Remember that I mentioned earlier that no cycle is the same and is different for every woman. There is no such thing as a 'right' cycle, except what is right for you.

So, take back your power to know yourself and begin to track your own cycles and rhythm. Notice how you feel and what you need in each of your seasons. Perhaps pay attention to where you are pushing and not honouring yourself during certain times of the month, and notice whether honouring your inner seasons and the feminine archetypes shift things for you.

There are several different apps that you can use to track this or begin a journal specifically for menstrual cycle awareness where you journal each day on your energy, moods, needs and where you are in your cycle.

The Moon and Menstruation

Even though there have never really been any in-depth studies on it, for a long time the link between the moon and women's menstrual cycles has been dismissed, ignored, denied and debated. For me, the two are inextricably linked. I truly believe that our ancestors would have bled in rhythm with the moon and agree with the suggestion that artificial lights and our modern-day lifestyles have lessened our connection to the moon, and her influence on our natural cycles.

The term 'menstruation' originates from the Latin word *mensis*, which means month and the Greek word *mene*, which means moon. The average woman's cycle is the same length as the average lunar cycle, approximately 29 days, and, during this time, women, just like the moon, go through several different phases.

Through the ages, the moon has been linked to the feminine and fertility, and we too can begin to look at where we bleed in relation to the moon and harness her wisdom and power alongside our own. Remember that your cycle can and will switch between these different cycles and there is no one cycle that is right or any better than the other. What's important is paying attention to your cycles and their messages, and honouring them in the best way for you.

The white moon cycle

Traditionally, women would have bled with the new moon and ovulated on the full moon. This is known as a white moon cycle and mirrors the cycle of the moon, going inwards and retreating when the moon retreats from the sky, and being at your most fertile when the moon is full in the sky.

When you bleed in this way, you are being asked to care for yourself and listen to your inner world, using the dark/new moon and your bleed to slow all the way down and access your feminine wisdom and deep emotional intelligence.

This is a fertile cycle indicating the creation of something, whether that is a readiness to become a mother and create life or a new project. As you mirror the moon, she takes you into the darkness to your inner hopes, dreams and desires, and assists you in bringing them to life through the following lunar cycle. However, that creation can only come through rest and stillness, and, if you bleed in this way, your big lesson is in surrender and receiving. The new moon and your period are not a time for doing but resting, retreating and gathering what you need. The more you can do this, the more you'll be at the peak of your energy and ready to create and shine during your ovulation and the full moon.

The pink moon cycle

This is when you bleed during the waxing moon – the moon's journey from new to full as she gets bigger and brighter in the sky every night. This is a cycle of growth, which indicates that you are in a transitional journey in your own life, on your way somewhere towards something.

This is a cycle for acting and making things happen in your life, exploring new possibilities and moving in a new direction. Use the wisdom of your bleed to discover more of yourself and guide you on how you can put yourself out there into the world, expanding into more of who you want to be.

The red moon cycle

The red moon cycle is when you bleed with the full moon and ovulate during the new moon. This is the cycle of the priestess, witches, healers and medicine women. These would have been the women who, at their peak ovulating energy, would have cared for and tended to the other women in the red tent or moon lodge (see page 216).

When you bleed in this way, you are being asked to use the wisdom and knowing that comes with your bleed, combined with the illuminating power of the full moon, to offer something out there to the world. Use the time of your bleed to focus on what you are being asked to create, offer and share with the world or how you can make the biggest difference to those around you.

Rather than self-care, this cycle is focused on self-development, using the quieter days of the dark moon as you are ovulating to dive deep into how you can grow, develop and evolve. This is a time for studying, self-enquiry, self-understanding and harnessing the power of the full moon to show you what you need to know.

This is a cycle of magic, mysticism, healing and reconnecting to your inner priestess and medicine woman to show you the gifts, experiences and wisdom that you have to offer that need to be shared. You are being called to step more into your power during a red cycle.

The purple moon cycle

This is when you bleed between the full and new moon as the moon wanes and gets smaller in the sky each night. Once more, this symbolises a transitional journey in your own life, but this time focus on a deep release and shedding what is no longer honouring or serving you.

Use the wisdom of your bleed to show you what it's time to walk away from, how you need to honour yourself, your time and your energy more, and where you need more rest and time for yourself.

AFFIRMATIONS TO RECLAIM
SEASONS AND CYCLES

O 'I honour my inner seasons and cycles.'

O 'I no longer push against my natural flow.'

O 'I reclaim the power of my period.'

O 'I move to my own natural rhythm.'

O 'I listen to the wisdom within.'

Now you've reclaimed your inner seasons and cycles, you get to move to your own natural rhythm and, in doing so, fully honour the Goddess within. Let's take this inner knowing now and use it to reclaim your purpose.

'To know yourself is to know your purpose.'

Chapter 12

RECLAIM YOUR PURPOSE

We continue along the Goddess Path now towards reclaiming your purpose.

Discovering your purpose helps give you a sense of direction and meaning in life and a reason for why you do what you do. It becomes a motivating force and helps you to feel like you are contributing to the world in a meaningful way, which is something that we all ultimately want to feel.

Living a life of purpose is essential to wellbeing and is one of the most soulful and heart-led ways to live. I also believe that finding and living your purpose is part of why you exist, it's part of why you're here, and you and your purpose is needed in the world.

We've all likely questioned our purpose at times, and even whether we have one. Perhaps we've believed that if we could only find our purpose we'd be happy/fulfilled/able to be who we want to be (fill in the gap). How to find purpose is one of the things I am asked about the most.

We often think of purpose as some elusive thing outside of us that we are constantly searching for. Yet it always feels just out of reach, and we never seem to find it, leaving us feeling lost, empty and directionless. We tend to look to the outside world to give our lives purpose and meaning, and, in doing so, lose ourselves even more. Or we think our purpose must be this big, life-changing thing that means we need to give up everything, quit our jobs and run off to India to become a yoga teacher. Although for some people that calling may be true (hello me!), that's not the same for everyone.

We also often fall into the trap of thinking that our purpose must be our job, and in many instances that may be true, but not necessarily. The likelihood is that the more you begin to realise, know and trust your purpose, the more you will feel naturally called to share that with the world. But your job is equally allowed to simply be a job, a place you go to work and earn money, and your purpose can live outside of that. You can find a purpose, a calling, without receiving a pay cheque for it by contributing to your family, community and all those you come into contact with in a way that only you can.

Because the truth is, and this is a big spoiler alert, your purpose is YOU. You are your purpose. There is no one else in the world like you. No one else who can do things the way you do them or share things the way you share them or say things the way you say them. Your main purpose in this world is to simply be more you. That's it. Your soul didn't come here to be anyone else; it came here to be you and bring what only you can offer.

For some people, their purpose is to be a stay-at-home mum raising the next generation of brilliant humans. For others, it's to be an office manager and, through managing people in a compassionate, loving and kind way, they get to change the lives of not only the people who work for them, but also their friends' and families' lives as they are more happy, secure and confident in their job, and this filters out into their home lives. Your purpose may be to be the best listener to those around you, shaping their lives by the fact they feel heard, held and understood. It may be to share your experiences so that others know they aren't alone or to share the wisdom of your experiences to help others around you. It may be to do your own healing work so as not to continue to repeat cycles and patterns. It may be to fight for social causes or to bring as much joy as you can into the lives of those around you.

After following the Goddess Path almost to the end, I really hope that you now know your value, worth and what you have to offer to the world, just by being you. I hope that you have reclaimed and set your inner Goddess free and that you know and trust yourself like never before. I hope that you are now ready to reclaim your purpose and begin to offer the world what only you can offer: YOU. Because we need you, the world needs you and what you have to offer.

Let's look at some ways that you can do that now . . .

To Know Yourself Is to Know Your Purpose

As we've seen, your purpose isn't something outside of you – it's already there, within you. You can't possibly begin to know your purpose if you don't know yourself. So spend time with yourself, know yourself, reflect on what makes you uniquely you, what you have to offer to the world and what you are called to share, and then begin to share you with everyone around you. The more you can be you and offer you to the world, the more your purpose will become clear.

Get honest about whether you are showing up as all of you in day-to-day life or whether you are still shrinking and dimming parts of yourself, holding back your truth or living out of alignment with your values in certain areas of your life. When you can begin to show up in your fullest presence and authenticity, you will start to feel more purposeful and alive.

Go inwards and feel what the Goddess wants to weave and create and bring to life through you – what are you most passionate about, what is most alive within you, what are you good at or knowledgeable about, what life experiences do you have that you could share to help and support others?

Every dream and desire within you is part of your purpose – they are in there for you to bring to life. I truly believe that we are never given a dream without also being given the means to achieve it, but they too are buried within and need to be discovered and uncovered as you allow yourself to grow into more of the Goddess that you came here to be.

You came here for a reason. Each and every one of us is here on purpose and the world just wouldn't be the same without you in it. So, it's your job not to hide and deny the world of your purpose, but to know that your purpose is to be you and begin to offer all that you are and have to the world.

Reclamation ritual

For the next week, live your life as though you are completely on purpose. As though every conversation you have is on purpose, every interaction you have is on purpose, every challenge that comes along is on purpose, every action you take is on purpose, every decision you make is on purpose, every day you wake up is on purpose.

How would that feel – to really feel as though you are on purpose? Because you are; your whole life is your purpose. See what shifts this week by believing in that fully and completely.

Make Your Whole Life Your Purpose

It's important to realise that your purpose can and will change over your lifetime as you evolve and grow as a person. For example, my various purposes have been to be a crystal healer, a yoga teacher, a moon mentor and an author, to name just a few, and each one of these purposes has kept leading me to even more purpose.

You will likely have many 'little' purposes in your life too, such as healing ancestral trauma, or teaching someone in your life something, or raising a family, or making a difference in the business/industry/company you work for, or helping someone else in your life heal. For now, your personal growth and walking the Goddess Path may be your purpose, as it's teaching you more about who you are, what you want and what you can offer.

The only way to fulfil your purpose and keep being given more of your soul mission is to keep growing into and becoming more of you. If you want to have a big purpose in life, you need to keep growing and evolving into the version of you who can hold that purpose.

When I knew I wanted to go to India and be a yoga teacher, it took me nearly two years to get there. I locked myself in the toilets of my corporate job and cried every day about why my dream wasn't coming true. But I now know that had I gone two years earlier, I wouldn't be sitting here writing this book for you now. I wasn't ready. My soul knew that there were still things I needed to learn and ways I needed to grow and evolve to be ready for the next part of my journey. And so, my purpose at that time was to keep studying, deepening my faith and trust in the universe, practising yoga, working more deeply with Goddess energy, crystals, manifesting, creative visualisation, meditating and praying. I didn't see it at the time, but all these things were leading me to this moment and to my purpose right now. I use all these tools in my life and teaching, and have decades of experience embodying these things so that I can now share them with you.

You may look at me and say, 'Well, it's all right for you, you know and are living your purpose' and yes I am. But it's taken me decades of little purposes and growing into the purpose that you see before you right now. So, begin to see everything that happens in your life as holding purpose for you and a way to learn and grow and get closer to the Goddess. Even if you are currently 'stuck' in a corporate job that you know isn't your purpose, how can you learn and grow as a human and soul through this experience? How can you still bring more of you and your purpose to your workplace and show up, speak up, be seen and allow yourself to be guided by the Goddess?

Your purpose is not some short-term quick life fix that you will discover one day and your whole life will change. Rather, your life will change when you begin to live as though your entire life is on purpose, as I suggested in the reclamation ritual above. The more you can do this, the more you'll begin to realise that all these little purposes are taking you somewhere closer to living your deeper purpose. The Goddess has a plan for you; all you need to do is trust her and go with her flow.

Reclamation ritual

Take some time to identify all the little purposes in your life that have brought you to this point. Journal on what each one was, what it taught you, how it helped you to discover or grow into more of yourself and how it's brought you here, to this moment. Then, begin to explore how you, at this time in your life, are being called to step into more of your purpose – what could your purpose be right now? What can you study, learn or do differently this week that may take you towards your purpose? Remember that it's very unlikely that any of us wake up one day and land in our exact purpose – we need to go through those little purposes first as we explore and uncover more of our deeper purpose.

For example, if you've always had an interest in life coaching, do a course. You may not ever end up becoming a life coach, but the journey towards that may open you up to more of your purpose. Everything you do that makes you more you and expands your knowing and wisdom is taking you further along your Goddess Path and leading you into more purpose.

Trust and Follow Your Purpose

This is the scary part, and the part that many people don't want to do, and so they wait for that elusive purpose to land on their doorstep (which it rarely ever does). You have to trust, follow and live your purpose, as this is part of expanding into it. If you have something to say, say it. If you have something to share, share it. If you get an intuitive niggle to do something, do it. It may not make total sense at the time, but intuition and purpose tend not to as they're part of the journey of trust and discovery that leads you to more purpose.

You may get a little inner nudge to begin to take care of your health and yourself, which may eventually lead to you sharing your journey and creating a business around helping others to do the same. You may feel an overwhelming urge to own your own power and strength and speak up for yourself or be brave enough to leave a relationship that's not working, and others will see this and be inspired enough to be able to do the same for themselves. You may even end up coaching and supporting other women in similar situations.

There may be the little voice that tells you that there are so many other people already doing what you want to do, that you don't know enough or do enough to make a difference in the world, that it's not the right time or you'll wait until this, that or then – and this is showing you what will always hold you back if you allow it to. Because honestly, there may be hundreds of other people doing what you want to do, but none of them will do it like you. I've been working with the moon for nearly 15 years, long before it became as popular as it is now. And when I first started sharing the life-changing work of Lunar Living, I was often ridiculed and rubbished, and not many people were listening. But I just couldn't not share it – it was, and still is, part of my purpose and something in me made me keep going, and I'm so glad that I did.

Reclamation rituals

Find more of your purpose daily

Find the feeling of your purpose, or its essence or your why, and then do more of that daily. What makes you feel most on purpose? Is it to help people, to create change, to be a leader, to talk to people, to invent something, to be a voice for those who don't have one, to work with children, to be on stage, to raise women, to write, to share your passion for numbers or crystals or music? Whatever it is, begin to do more of that in your everyday life with the people you already have around you.

Write a 'life experience CV'

Rather than the standard CV that lists education and jobs, I want you to write one that lists your life experiences and all that you have learned. Write down anything and everything that makes you 'qualified' to be you and to share your purpose with the world. List all your natural gifts and talents, as well as the key turning points, learning curves and challenges, and all that you have overcome.

Journal on purpose

Journal each day on how you are already inspiring everyone around you – how your words, presence, advice, wisdom, teachings and you just being you and showing up in your Goddess presence is inspiring everyone you come into contact with.

INVOKE THE GODDESS

Brigid is the Celtic Goddess of spring, fertility, magic, healing, clairvoyance and divination. She is considered a triple Goddess, with three roles or purposes: Goddess of healing waters, Goddess of the sacred flame and Goddess of fertile earth.

Her name means 'exalted one', 'fiery arrow' or 'bright one' and, as such, she helps you to begin to see and step into your full potential, grow into all that you can be, allow yourself to begin to shine brightly and to aim for what you want.

A Goddess of wisdom and inspiration, she will help you to uncover your unique gifts and talents, and encourage you to begin to share them with those around you and the world. She brings abundance, fertility, vital life force energy and new beginnings, helping you to realise and actualise the seeds of the dreams within you and bring them into reality.

Wash away your doubts

As the keeper of sacred springs and healing wells, Brigid will help you to heal and wash away all the doubts and fears that prevent you from knowing and stepping into your full purpose. When you notice yourself in a spiral of not believing you have anything to offer or holding yourself back, take a ritual bath or shower. You could even visit the sea, a lake or a stream if you have them nearby. As you immerse yourself in the water, call on Brigid and ask her to wash away your doubts and feel her healing waters cleanse you of your fears.

Tend to your own inner flame

Close your eyes. Call on Brigid and let her show you the flame of purpose that burns within you. This is the divine spark of life force energy that is unique to you and only you. Each day, with Brigid's help, visualise this flame within you and see it growing bigger and shining more brightly. Allow the light of this sacred flame to start to fill your entire body so that you begin to radiate and shine your inner purpose. Anytime you feel your flame is dim, think about how you can tend to it and bring more light to your purpose flame.

> ### Nurture your purpose seeds
>
> Visualise little seeds of purpose that have been planted within you that only you can bring to life. What do these seeds need to grow and come to life? When you plant physical seeds, you need to water, fertilise and perhaps repot them, make sure they are getting enough light and do all you can to help them to grow. Do the same for your inner seeds. Call on Brigid to help you to keep your inner world fertile and ensure that you are giving yourself the right conditions to grow into your most purposeful self.

Embody the Archetypes

The queen

Call on your inner queen to help you to know that you are here on purpose and have something valuable to offer to the world, just by being you. Let her show you how to claim your rightful place of purpose in the world.

The priestess

Let your inner priestess teach you how to be in deep devotion to yourself, and in turn your purpose. She will help you to trust the guidance that is leading you forwards towards your path of purpose.

Pray For Your Purpose

Begin each day with a prayer for purpose. Find your own words for what feels right for you, but ask to be shown how you can make more of a difference and be more on purpose. Ask that the universe and the Goddess flow through you and use you in the very best ways to make the greatest difference in the world. Or just simply ask, 'How can I be of service?' as often as you can. This is your purpose – to be of service and to be more you.

AFFIRMATIONS TO RECLAIM YOUR PURPOSE

- ○ 'I am my purpose.'
- ○ 'My purpose is to be me.'
- ○ 'My purpose becomes clearer every day.'
- ○ 'I am always being guided towards more purpose.'
- ○ 'I live a purposeful life.'
- ○ 'I make a difference every day.'

I truly hope that, through this chapter, you now know that your only purpose is to allow the world the gift of more you. We need you, just as the Goddess that you are. It's time now to reclaim YOU.

'You are the Goddess that we all need. You are the Goddess you have been waiting for.'

Chapter 13

RECLAIM YOU

So here we are my Loves, at the end of the Goddess Path. I truly hope that this has been an enlightening journey of self-discovery, self-awareness, self-exploration and, most of all, reclamation and remembering of all of who you are. It's time now to reintroduce yourself to the world and remerge as the true Goddess you came here to be.

I truly believe that one of the biggest compliments someone can give us is 'you've changed'. Usually meant as an insult, it is in fact confirmation that we are evolving, growing and becoming in the way that we are supposed to on our journey of life. We don't come here to stay the same, remain stuck in our comfort zones and live under the weight of other people's opinions and expectations. We come here to discover who we are and what part and purpose we have to play in the ever-unfolding world that we are part of.

I hope that you have changed on your journey along the Goddess Path. I hope that you can look back to who you were when you started this journey and hold this version of you with such tenderness for all she was about to discover about herself. Take some time now to reflect on your journey. Look back to who you were at the beginning. Perhaps write her a letter of all the things that you would like to tell her. Look at the lessons, challenges, growth, tears, joys, highs, lows and everything in between. Really take some time here to process, celebrate and integrate your journey.

If I was to ask you now, at the end of this journey, who you are, what would you tell me? In Chapter 2 I told you that, 'By the end of this book, I want you to be able to tell me who you are. I want you to be able to tell me of your greatness, your worth and your purpose. I want you to be able to tell me of your values, your hopes and dreams and desires, your wildness, your shadows, what you're good at, what makes you happy, what you can bring to the world and everything that makes up the very essence of you.'

I truly hope that you can tell me all of that now.

The most exciting news of all is that it doesn't end here – this is just the very beginning. You are only just getting started and, as you invite more of the Goddess into your life and show up as more of her, your life will only get better and better.

Let's look at some ways now to keep the magic alive as you go back out there into the world and take this magical, life-changing work with you.

INVOKE THE GODDESS

The Goddess that we now call upon is **you**. To show up and be seen and shine in the world and offer what only you can. You are the Goddess that we all need. But if you are ever in any doubt, know that you have a whole team of Goddesses right beside you, both seen and unseen, cheering you on.

Going forwards, begin to live as the Goddess. Visualise your inner Goddess, the divine feminine energy that wants to weave and create things in the world through you. Envision yourself as her, feel her and begin to move through the world as her. Walk down the street as the Goddess, do your supermarket shop as the Goddess, go to your work meetings as the Goddess, pick up your children from school as the Goddess, begin to live your life as her.

See if every now and then you can live an entire day dedicated to the Goddess, where you allow the divine feminine to flow through your day completely. That may mean an 11am start as Shakti wants a slow start to the morning or a 2pm bath as Shakti wants to luxuriate in bubbles. Eat your food slowly and savour every mouthful, drink your morning coffee as though it's the best thing you've ever experienced. Invite as much pleasure and flow into your day as you can and just follow the Goddess to wherever she wants to guide you.

Reclamation ritual

Reintroduce yourself. Who are you now? What do you want, need, desire and believe? How are you committed to showing up in the world as all of you? What is your truth, your purpose, your offering? What are you no longer accepting or allowing? What are you inviting in and embracing?

This is the moment when you get to reclaim your full Goddess power and re-emerge into the world as all of who you came here to be. Do that now. Journal on who you now are at the end of this journey and make yourself some promises and commitments of how you will begin to show up in the world as more of the Goddess that you are and how you will continue to keep this journey alive.

Perhaps do a future-self visualisation, where you envision yourself in six months' time. With your new-found self-belief and knowing what you are now capable of, see everything you want to have created in your life by then and who you are growing into.

Now, begin to become her in your day-to-day life. How would this future-self Goddess version of you speak, think, act, behave and show up in the world? Begin to embody her, grow into her, become her. Call upon the Goddesses and your sisters when you need them; know you don't need to do this journey alone.

AFFIRMATIONS TO RECLAIM YOU

- ◯ 'I am the Goddess that the world has been waiting for.'
- ◯ 'I reclaim my full Goddess power.'
- ◯ 'I let my full self be seen and shine.'
- ◯ 'I embody, grow into and become the Goddess.'
- ◯ 'I live as the Goddess.'
- ◯ 'I allow the divine feminine energy to weave and create things through me.'

THANK YOU

Thank you so much for taking this journey. For allowing me to be your guide along this path. For being brave enough to dive into your depths and reclaim the Goddess within. I need you, we need you, the world needs you in your full Goddess power and magic.

I have tears streaming down my face writing these closing words as I am so incredibly proud of you, your journey and all that is yet to come for you. You have no idea the difference you make in the world just by being you and how many people you will inspire through walking the Goddess Path.

I truly hope you now know how special, beautiful, purposeful, powerful and deserving you are. You are a Goddess, and don't you ever forget that. And if you ever do, both the Goddesses and I are here to remind you.

Please share your journey and experiences along the Goddess Path with me, tagging me on Instagram (@kirsty_gallagher_). I always love to hear from you.

From the bottom of my heart, thank you.

GODDESS GLOSSARY

Aphrodite: Goddess of love, beauty, fertility, prosperity and desire, she teaches you the art of self-love and receiving.

Artemis: Goddess of the moon, nature and the wilds, she teaches you how to embody and embrace your emotions.

Athena: Goddess of war and wisdom, she will bring you strength, power and courage when you need it the most.

Brigid: Goddess of spring, the healing waters, sacred flame and fertile earth, she will help you to see your full potential and grow into all that you can be.

Ceridwen: Keeper of the cauldron of knowledge, transformation and change, she is the Goddess to call upon when you are ready to change and transform.

Durga: Warrior Goddess of protection and strength, she is the one to call upon when you need to access the true source of your inner power and knowing.

Ereshkigal: Goddess of the underworld, she will help you to go into deep self-reflection and discovery of the depths of your inner world and all that you have hidden to see the truth of who you are.

Gaia: Goddess of the earth and ancestral mother of all life, she provides anchoring, stability and safety.

Hecate: Queen of the witches, magic, crossroads, the night and the moon, she will help you to set boundaries and find your way when you are lost.

Isis: The great healer and Goddess of magic and protection, she will help you to explore past lives and awaken your innate healing powers.

Kali: Goddess of time, life, death, creation and destruction, she helps you to release attachments, take back your power and transform your life.

Lilith: A Dark Goddess representing rebellion, freedom, independence and feminine empowerment, she is the Goddess to call upon when you have lost yourself or need to express your true self.

Maat: Goddess of wisdom, truth and cosmic order, she will help you to find your voice and speak your truth from within.

The Morrigan: A shape-shifting triple Goddess, the Morrigan will help you to face your deepest fears and uncover any parts of you that you have buried in shame.

Nyx: Goddess of the night and the darkness, Nyx will help you to face your fears, uncover your deepest truths and stay safe in the darkness, no longer fearing the shadows.

Oshun: Goddess of femininity, fertility and sensuality, she will teach you how to flow with life and awaken your creativity and sensuality.

Persephone: Goddess of springtime, Persephone spends half the year in the underworld. She will teach you how to embrace your shadows without losing your light and how to stay true to yourself.

Ragana: Goddess of witchcraft, she will help you to stop hiding and reveal more of your true self to the world.

Rhiannon: Goddess of healing, transformation and rebirth, she brings strength and courage and teaches us forgiveness.

Saraswati: Goddess of flow, expression and feminine wisdom, she will help you to awaken your creativity and intuition.

Venus: Similar to her Greek sister Aphrodite, she will teach you of your values, self-worth and how to care for yourself.

ENDNOTES

1   Mental Health Foundation, 14 May 2018. "Stressed nation: 74% of UK 'overwhelmed or unable to cope' at some point in the past year." Retrieved from https://www.mentalhealth.org. uk/about-us/news/survey-stressed-nation-UK-overwhelmed-unable-to-cope; CIPHR, n.d. "Workplace stress statistics in the UK." Retrieved from https://www.ciphr.com/workplace-stress-statistics/; Bowling, G., 7 Oct. 2022. "Why women are more at risk of burnout." Nuffield Health. Retrieved from https://www. nuffieldhealth.com/article/why-women-are-more-at-risk-of-burnout.

2   Rodriguez, L., 9 Oct. 2020. "When will accurate period ads stop getting banned?" Global Citizen. Retrieved from https:// www.globalcitizen.org/en/content/facebook-banned-modi bodi-period-ad/; Harvey-Jenner, C., 17 Oct. 2017. "The first ever advert showing period blood has arrived." *Cosmopolitan.* Retrieved from https://www.cosmopolitan.com/uk/reports/ a13034226/bodyform-advert-first-show-period-blood/.

ACKNOWLEDGEMENTS

To my wonderful family: Sandra, Kylie, Kerry, Liam, Stephanie, Soraya, Jake, Chloe, Edward, Isaac and my late Grandpa Donald. I love you all and thank you for always loving and supporting me.

To Sam, you're my person. Thank you for always walking alongside me and for your endless support and encouragement, and to my godson Harley and my Welsh family, thank you.

Thank you to Holly Whitaker, I love making books with you. Thank you for always believing in me. Thank you to my new Ebury family, I am so excited for this journey together. Special mentions to Alice Gordge and Ellie Crisp for all your hard work and support, and to Mylène Mozas-Sauvignon for creating such a beautiful front cover.

To my copyeditor Julia Kellaway, thank you for such thoughtful and helpful edits and for making the process easy and enjoyable. Thanks too to Alex Cameron for your beautiful photographs and the WillCarne team for your videos.

Thank you to Fearne Cotton (and your brilliant family) for your friendship and support and to Happy Place for having me as part of the family. I love contributing to the app and festivals and now making books with you too.

To my northern sister Melanie C, thank you for being you and for your support and friendship.

To the Goddess, this would not be possible without you. Thank you for weaving your magic through my life and guiding me along my journey. This is for you.

If you are holding this book in your hands, thank you for allowing me to share the wisdom of the Goddesses with you. I truly hope this book guides you on a journey of self-discovery to reclaiming your most intuitive, authentic and powerful self. I always love to hear from you so please do share your Goddess magic with me.

To my Lunar Living online sisterhood, thank you for all your support, lunar love and for being the best sisterhood ever. My never-ending gratitude to my right-hand woman Helen Elias, nothing I do would be what it is without you.

Thank you to everyone in my IG and online community. You are the most supportive and magical community ever. Thank you for continuing to show up for yourself and each other. Remember, you are never alone, you've got this, I've got you, we've got each other. We're only just getting started and there is so much yet to come.

Thank you to Chris Evans, Tash and family for your support and friendship, and to everyone on the *Breakfast Show* and CarFest team for allowing me to share the moon magic and my work with the nation. I love you all.

Thanks too to *This Morning*, Mind Body Spirit, Peligoni, Stylist Warehouse, *You* magazine, *Red* magazine, *Happiful* magazine and everyone who has invited me on your podcasts or lives to share my work. Thank you to Zoe and Morgan for your magical jewellery.

Special mentions to these special people in my life, you know who you are and what you do: Becki Rabin, Julie Morrow, Brett Waters, Lisa Strong, my Costa Rica witches Soulla and Lyah, Rebecca Dennis, Rangan and Vidh Chatterje, Caggie Dunlop and Ian Steed.

If I have not named you, it's not because you are forgotten or that I am not grateful. It's simply that I have been blessed to have so many wonderful people touch my life and not enough pages left to mention you all, it would be another book in itself! If you have ever been a part of my life in any way, thank you.

ABOUT THE AUTHOR

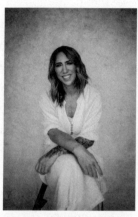

Photograph by Alexandra Cameron

Kirsty Gallagher is the UK's leading voice in spirituality. She is a moon mentor, soul alignment and spiritual coach, yoga teacher, meditation teacher and *Sunday Times* bestselling author. She teaches you how to live back in alignment with your soul and divine purpose by reconnecting with ancient wisdoms and natural cycles.

Kirsty is renowned worldwide for her deep and innate knowledge of the divine feminine, Goddess energy, lunar cycles and astrology, living by the seasons, crystals, meditation and yoga. Her book titles include the *Sunday Times* bestseller *Lunar Living, The Lunar Living Journal, Crystals for Self-Care* and *Sacred Seasons*.

Kirsty has been sharing the life-changing benefits of her work for over 20 years through classes, workshops and events, and has taught at more than 80 worldwide retreats. She is the founder of the growing online sisterhood *Lunar Living*, which connects women from all over the world and teaches them how to weave the wisdom of the moon into everyday, modern life.

Kirsty works alongside women from all walks of life teaching them how to live back in alignment with a natural rhythm and flow, helping them to connect back to their inner wisdom, power, authenticity and purpose.

Weaving lunar, nature and Goddess wisdom with spiritual teachings, astrology and her unique and transformative mentoring, Kirsty helps women to step into their power by overcoming doubts, fears and self-sabotage. She invites them to live boldly and unapologetically, and to know and trust in themselves like never before to find greater meaning and purpose in life.

Kirsty has created an engaged worldwide community through her popular online and in-person events and social media platforms, where she shares her unique insights and wisdom of ancient practices and mysticism. Her greatest passion is bringing together community and showing us that we are never alone. She has become a guiding light for women around the globe who seek out her beautifully delivered guidance on navigating their spiritual paths intertwined with busy, modern-day lives.

Kirsty is a sought-after and leading voice in spiritual and soul-led personal development, having regularly featured on *The Chris Evans Breakfast Show* and *This Morning*; is a contributor on Fearne Cotton's *Happy Place App* and *Happy Place* festivals, and has been featured in *YOU, Stylist, Red, Women's Health, Soul & Spirit* and *Natural Health* magazines.

Described as personable, down-to-earth, compassionate, warm-hearted and inspiring, Kirsty is known for delivering her life-changing and unmatched knowledge of ancient wisdoms in an easy-to-understand and relatable way that anyone and everyone can take something from.

Find out more at kirstygallagher.com or join her Instagram community at @kirsty_gallagher_.

NOTES

NOTES

NOTES

NOTES

NOTES

NOTES